Wolf Blecher

The Hilbert-Moore Sequence

Wolf Blecher

The Hilbert-Moore Sequence

Acoustic Noise Optimized MR Imaging

Südwestdeutscher Verlag für Hochschulschriften

Impressum/Imprint (nur für Deutschland/ only for Germany)
Bibliografische Information der Deutschen Nationalbibliothek: Die Deutsche Nationalbibliothek
verzeichnet diese Publikation in der Deutschen Nationalbibliografie; detaillierte bibliografische
Daten sind im Internet über http://dnb.d-nb.de abrufbar.

Alle in diesem Buch genannten Marken und Produktnamen unterliegen warenzeichen-, marken-
oder patentrechtlichem Schutz bzw. sind Warenzeichen oder eingetragene Warenzeichen der
jeweiligen Inhaber. Die Wiedergabe von Marken, Produktnamen, Gebrauchsnamen,
Handelsnamen, Warenbezeichnungen u.s.w. in diesem Werk berechtigt auch ohne besondere
Kennzeichnung nicht zu der Annahme, dass solche Namen im Sinne der Warenzeichen- und
Markenschutzgesetzgebung als frei zu betrachten wären und daher von jedermann benutzt
werden dürften.

Verlag: Südwestdeutscher Verlag für Hochschulschriften Aktiengesellschaft & Co. KG
Dudweiler Landstr. 99, 66123 Saarbrücken, Deutschland
Telefon +49 681 37 20 271-1, Telefax +49 681 37 20 271-0, Email: info@svh-verlag.de
Zugl.: Mannheim, Universität, Diss., 2008

Herstellung in Deutschland:
Schaltungsdienst Lange o.H.G., Berlin
Books on Demand GmbH, Norderstedt
Reha GmbH, Saarbrücken
Amazon Distribution GmbH, Leipzig
ISBN: 978-3-8381-0591-8

Imprint (only for USA, GB)
Bibliographic information published by the Deutsche Nationalbibliothek: The Deutsche
Nationalbibliothek lists this publication in the Deutsche Nationalbibliografie; detailed
bibliographic data are available in the Internet at http://dnb.d-nb.de.

Any brand names and product names mentioned in this book are subject to trademark, brand or
patent protection and are trademarks or registered trademarks of their respective holders. The
use of brand names, product names, common names, trade names, product descriptions etc.
even without a particular marking in this works is in no way to be construed to mean that such
names may be regarded as unrestricted in respect of trademark and brand protection legislation
and could thus be used by anyone.

Publisher:
Südwestdeutscher Verlag für Hochschulschriften Aktiengesellschaft & Co. KG
Dudweiler Landstr. 99, 66123 Saarbrücken, Germany
Phone +49 681 37 20 271-1, Fax +49 681 37 20 271-0, Email: info@svh-verlag.de

Copyright © 2009 by the author and Südwestdeutscher Verlag für Hochschulschriften
Aktiengesellschaft & Co. KG and licensors
All rights reserved. Saarbrücken 2009

Printed in the U.S.A.
Printed in the U.K. by (see last page)
ISBN: 978-3-8381-0591-8

Contents

1. **Introduction**   1
   1.1. Motivation 1
   1.2. Outline 2
   1.3. Technical Environment 2

2. **Magnetic Resonance Imaging - The Very Basics**   3
   2.1. Signal Generation 4
      2.1.1. Spin Basics 4
      2.1.2. Excitation & Relaxation 5
   2.2. Image encoding 8
      2.2.1. Slice Selection 8
      2.2.2. Phase- and Frequency Encoding 9
   2.3. Signal Echo Generation 10
   2.4. k-Space Formalism 10

3. **Trajectory Design**   15
   3.1. Common Trajectories 15
      3.1.1. FLASH 15
      3.1.2. Echo Planar Imaging 17
   3.2. Space Filling Curves 20
      3.2.1. History and Overview 20
      3.2.2. Hilbert's Space Filling Curve 22
      3.2.3. Space Filling Curves In Magnetic Resonance 24
   3.3. Trajectory Deviating Effects 26
   3.4. Implementation Of The Hilbert-Moore Sequence 29
      3.4.1. Design Considerations 29
      3.4.2. Gradient Amplitude Calculation 33

		3.5. Trajectory Verification	35
		3.6. Results	36
		3.6.1. Gradient Amplitudes	36
		3.6.2. Sequence Time Course	37
		3.6.3. Trajectory Deviation Simulation	38
		3.6.4. Trajectory Measurement	40
		3.7. Discussion	41

4. Image Reconstruction   44

- 4.1. Parallel Imaging 44
  - 4.1.1. SMASH 45
  - 4.1.2. PARS 46
  - 4.1.3. GRAPPA 47
  - 4.1.4. MCMLI 50
- 4.2. Hilbert-Moore Reconstruction 51
- 4.3. Results 53
  - 4.3.1. Simulation 53
  - 4.3.2. Scanner Phantom Data 59
- 4.4. Discussion 66

5. Sound   72

- 5.1. Implications 72
- 5.2. Sound Generation 74
- 5.3. Noise Reduction Mechanisms 74
  - 5.3.1. Hardware Modifications 75
  - 5.3.2. Imaging Strategies 76
  - 5.3.3. Acoustic Noise Optimizations for FLASH and EPI 77
- 5.4. Sound Measurement 77
  - 5.4.1. Equipment 78
  - 5.4.2. Microphone Calibration 78
  - 5.4.3. Measurement Setup 80
  - 5.4.4. Data Evaluation 80
- 5.5. Results 80
  - 5.5.1. Calibration 80

	5.5.2. Imaging Sequences	82
5.6.	Discussion	88

6. Summary   95
    6.1. Conclusion 95
    6.2. Outlook 96

A. Gradient encoding tables   99
    A.1. Replacement factors 99
    A.2. Gradient settings for VD center 99
    A.3. Gradient settings for HM trajectory 99

B. Calibration Sound Pressure Levels   102

This page has intentionally been left blank.

1. Introduction

1.1. Motivation

Over the last decades, Magnetic Resonance Imaging (MRI) has been experiencing a boom. The non-invasive imaging technique with its high contrast and image quality for soft tissues has become one of the standard diagnostic methods in medicine. The commercial availability of higher field strengths with even better image contrast every few years documents that MR is a field of ongoing research.

The variety of possible applications has led to the adoption of MR imaging to other sciences like psychology and neuro science. Especially functional MRI (fMRI) plays an important role in these two fields. Functional MRI can be used to show signal differences in certain brain regions during the fulfillment of tasks like finger-tapping, listening to sounds, enduring pain, and watching images or flickering patterns.

However, one disadvantage of MRI has not yet been mastered. During the acquisition of an image, the MR scanner emits a variety of sound noises, which reach sound pressure levels above the human pain threshold. This acoustic noise is not only a source of annoyance for the subject and the operator but can induce hearing damages and has certain influences on the results achieved by fMRI experiments.

Over the last ten years, several researchers have measured the acoustic noise generated by the MR imager and some improvements to reduce the acoustic noise by hardware modifications, different sampling strategies or optimizing imaging sequences have been proposed. None found its way into the commercial products.

In this work, a new imaging sequence based on the Hilbert-Moore space filling curve is developed which tackles the acoustic noise generated by the MR scanner from a different point of view. Instead of trying to suppress the acoustic noise generated during image acquisition, it is intended to shift the generated sound energy to acoustic frequencies above the human hearing threshold.

1.2. Outline

In chapter 2 the basic knowledge of MRI is explained using the classical model that does not involve quantum mechanics. The basics of signal generation and image encoding are explained as well as the theory of k-space.

Chapter 3 explains the design of the Hilbert-Moore imaging sequence. After a survey of existing imaging sequences, the necessary theory of space filling curves is shown. Finally, the design decisions met for the newly developed imaging sequence are explained and the resulting k-space trajectory is validated.

In chapter 4 the image reconstruction algorithm for the newly developed sequence is shown. A short introduction to parallel imaging with standard reconstruction algorithms that influenced the new reconstruction scheme is presented beforehand.

Chapter 5 leads back to the intention of this work, the reduction of the acoustic noise during MR imaging. A choice of hitherto existing attempts to reduce the acoustic noise is presented in combination with a description of the generation process of acoustic noise during MR imaging. The sound noise of the developed sequence is evaluated and compared to the sound noise of a standard imaging sequence.

Each chapter of this work is more or less self-contained. This means that each chapter (except the MRI basics in chapter 2) is organized into a introductory part, a methods and a results part followed by a short discussion. An individual bibliography concludes each chapter. The reason why I have chosen this approach is the independence of the different parts of the work. The sequence development covered in chapter 3 can be done without any knowledge of the reconstruction covered in chapter 4. The analysis of the sound noise needs the developed sequence but the methods and the theory of acoustic noise are completely independent of the methods and the theory of the other two parts.

1.3. Technical Environment

The new pulse sequence has been developed on a Siemens Tim TRIO 3T MR Imager (Siemens Medical, Erlangen) located at the Central Institute for Mental Health in Mannheim. The Siemens IDEA Software Framework version VB15 has been used for the development.

2. Magnetic Resonance Imaging - The Very Basics

The concept of Magnetic Resonance Imaging (MRI) can be brought down to a few simple steps:

1. Place a sample inside a magnetic field.

2. Irradiate with an electromagnetic (radio frequency) wave.

3. Acquire the signal generated by the sample.

4. Reconstruct the image by calculation of a Fourier transformation.

These steps are basically everything necessary to acquire an MR image. However, the theoretical background, based on quantum mechanics is more challenging than these four steps. In this chapter a general overview how MRI works in more detail than the four points given above is presented. The complete background (including quantum mechanics) is beyond the scope of this thesis. A Detailed introduction to the field of MRI in all its facets can be found in [1–3]. A very theoretical indepth introduction is given in [1]. The theoretical background and different facets of MR including (but not being limited to) spectroscopy, imaging in general, and flow imaging can be found in [2]. A very good introduction to MR pulse sequence development, the options and difficulties during design of a pulse sequence in addition to the necessary background theory for each decision to be made during the development process are described in [3].

The following introductory sections cover signal generation (section 2.1), position encoding (section 2.2) and signal echo generation (section 2.3). Section 2.4 presents the concept of k-space, that facilitates the understanding of pulse sequence trajectories and is thus inevitable for the rest of this work.

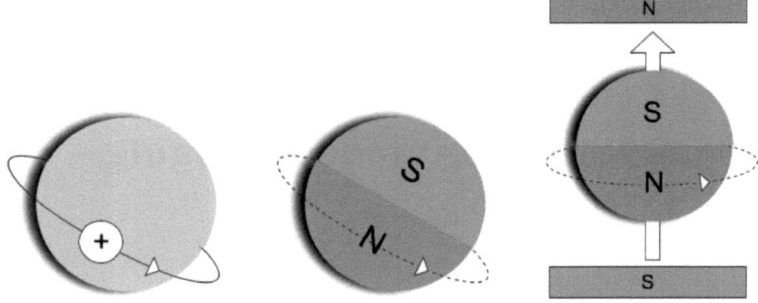

Figure 2.1.: *Schematic drawing of the proton spin*

Figure 2.2.: *Magnetic field induced by the proton spin*

Figure 2.3.: *Alignment with an external magnetic field*

2.1. Signal Generation

2.1.1. Spin Basics

Magnetic Resonance Imaging (MRI) is based on Nuclear Magnetic Resonance (NMR) spectroscopy which is widely used in chemistry and material science. The *nuclear* in NMR has nothing to do with nuclear in the sense of radioactivity but refers to the *nucleus* of an atom. The most basic atom is the hydrogen atom which has a single proton in its nucleus. Each proton has not only a positive charge but also a spin (like a planet e.g. the earth), depicted in figure 2.1. Each proton (due to mass and motion) can be assigned an angular momentum and a magnetic field. Thus, a proton can be compared to a small bar magnet, having a north and a south pole (figure 2.2). In the following, the rotating magnetization will also be referred to as *spin*.

If inserted into a larger (external) magnetic field, the proton will align with the magnetic field (2.3). This is the equilibrium state of the proton in an external magnetic field. If the equilibrium is disturbed (e.g. by inhomogeneities in the external magnetic field), the axis of the spin flips away from the main axis of the magnetic field and will precess around this main axis as shown in figure 2.4. An analogy is a spinning top being deviated from its upright rotation.

The precession frequency depends on the strength of the main magnetic field $\vec{B}$ (given in Tesla [T]) and on a spin dependent constant γ called the gyromagnetic ratio. For ^{1}H, γ equals 42.67 MHz/T. The precession (or Larmor) frequency ω can be calculated by

$$\omega = \gamma \cdot |\vec{B}|. \tag{2.1}$$

The common representation of the precession of the spin is a vector (representing the magnetization of the complete sample) and its position in a coordinate system, where the z-axis of the coordinate system points in the direction of the external magnetic field (figure 2.5)

To overcome the difficulty in calculations introduced by the precession of the magnetization vector, the *rotating reference frame* is introduced. Instead of respecting the precession of the magnetization in every calculation, it is assumed that the magnetization is immobile and the laboratory on the outside precesses. This changes the mathematics but not the physics. All following steps deal only with the magnetization vector and do not involve the outside laboratory. Thus, the rotating reference frame facilitates calculations and imagination. The coordinate system used in the subsequent parts of this thesis assumes the z-axis to be aligned with the main direction of the magnetization, and y- and x-axis being perpendicular to the z-axis (as depicted in figure 2.6).

2.1.2. Excitation & Relaxation

The equilibrium alignment of the samples magnetization in direction of the main magnetic field renders it impossible to distinguish the sample's magnetization and the main magnetic field. If the sample's magnetization could be flipped perpendicular to the main magnetic field it would be possible to measure it. The precession of the magnetization induces a current which is then acquired by a receive coil as the signal of the sample.

The necessary flip of the magnetization is achieved by irradiation of the sample with a radio frequency (RF) pulse with the resonance frequency of the sample. The angle α, by which the magnetization is flipped, is determined by the irradiation energy. The maximal signal is achieved if the energy transmitted by the RF pulse is adjusted to flip the magnetization by 90° to the x-y-plane. An RF pulse is usually referred by the flip angle of the magnetization. In figure 2.7(b) the effect of an pulse with flip angle $\alpha°$ is shown and figure 2.7(c) the effect of a 90° pulse is depicted.

2. Magnetic Resonance Imaging - The Very Basics

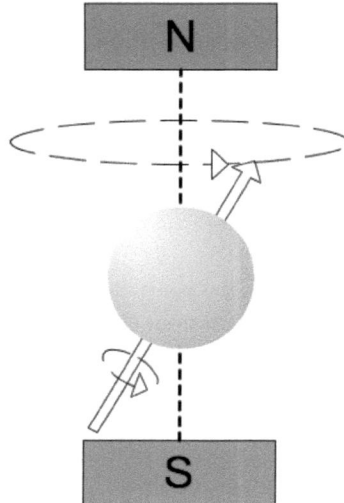

Figure 2.4.: *Precession of a proton around the axis of the main magnetic field*

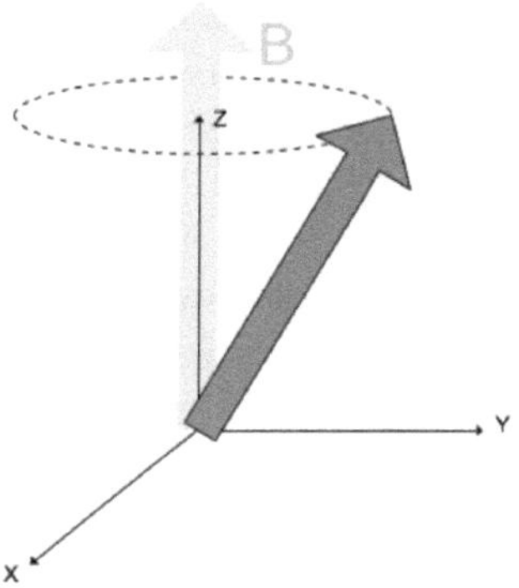

Figure 2.5.: *Coordinate system representation of the precessing magnetization*

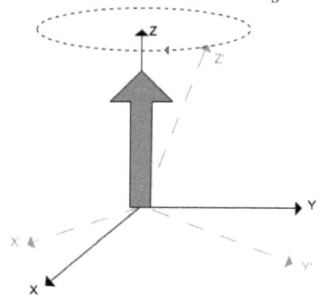

Figure 2.6.: *Immobile rotating reference frame and precessing laboratory coordinate frame (stippled gray, X', Y', Z' axes) as seen by the magnetization of the sample (red arrow)*

2. Magnetic Resonance Imaging - The Very Basics

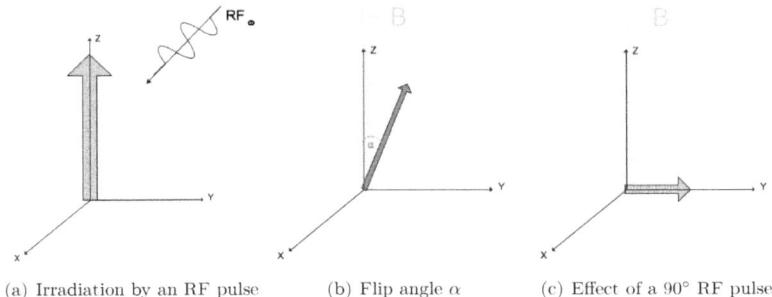

(a) Irradiation by an RF pulse (b) Flip angle α (c) Effect of a 90° RF pulse

Figure 2.7.: *Effect of an RF pulse. Figure (a) shows irradiation by an RF pulse with the same resonance frequency ω. Depending on the energy transmitted by the RF pulse, the magnetization is flipped by different angles exemplarily shown in (b) and (c)*

T_1 Relaxation

Once the magnetization has been flipped by an RF pulse to an energetically different state, it will return to the more favorable equilibrium state. This restoration of the longitudinal magnetization is called T_1 (or longitudinal) relaxation (figure 2.8). The energy consumed during the RF pulse is transferred to the environment. Depending on the environment (and as such on the sample) the time during which this process takes place is different but typically in the range of ~300 to 2000 ms.

T_2 Relaxation

In addition to the restoration of the longitudinal magnetization, the spins in the sample interact with each other. Due to these interactions, the transverse magnetization starts to decay once the RF pulse is switched off. A time constant T_2 is assigned to this process called T_2 (or transversal) relaxation. This relaxation process depends only on the spins and is therefore also called *spin-spin-relaxation*. Its typical time constant T_2 is in the range of ~30 to 150ms.

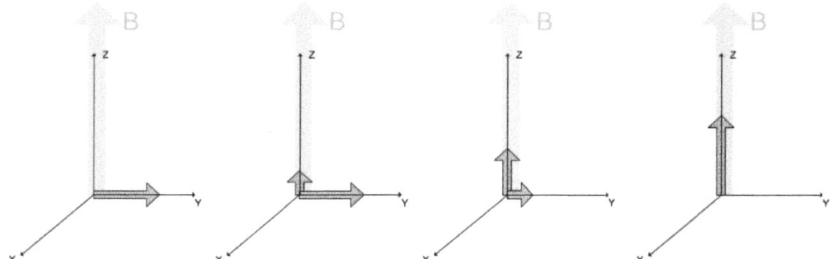

Figure 2.8.: T_1 *relaxation: More and more spins return to their initial state. This leads to a recreation of the longitudinal magnetization.*

T_2^* Relaxation

The reduction of the transverse magnetization does not only depend on (natural) T_2 relaxation but also on the homogeneity of the main magnetic field and other external factors. In contrast to the loss of the signal by T_1 and T_2 relaxation, the influence of these external factors can be revoked. This is used for the generation of a so called signal echo, explained in section 2.3.

2.2. Image encoding

In the previous section the generation of the signal has been described. Following these guidelines, a single frequency peak is observed instead of an image. The problem is that the whole sample experiences the same magnetic field and therefore all the spins in the sample have the same Larmor frequency. If an RF pulse with this frequency is switched on, the spins in the complete sample will be flipped and generate signal. In the following it is described how position is encoded during image acquisition.

2.2.1. Slice Selection

The main representation of MRI images is a 2D image which represents a thin slice (~2-10mm) of the object in the scanner. The first task during imaging is to select the slice i.e. excite solely the spins inside this slice and leave other spins in the sample

2. Magnetic Resonance Imaging - The Very Basics

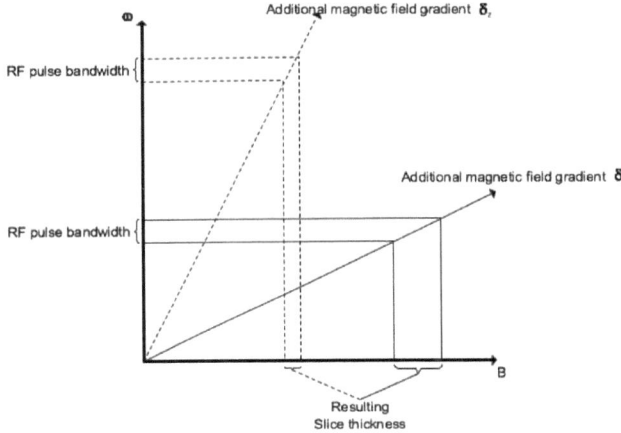

Figure 2.9.: *Relation between RF pulse bandwidth and resulting slice thickness. Depending on the gradient δ added to the B magnetic field, the same bandwidth leads to a different slice thickness.*

unaffected. This is solved by applying a linear magnetic field gradient in addition to the main magnetic field. Coming back to equation 2.1 the additional magnetic gradient changes the resonance (Larmor) frequency:

$$\omega = \gamma \cdot |\vec{B} + \vec{\delta}|. \tag{2.2}$$

The RF pulse is adjusted to irradiate not only a single frequency but a frequency range (it has a certain bandwidth). Only the spins with a Larmor frequency inside this range (defined by the additional gradient) get flipped, as shown in figure 2.9. This additional gradient conveys the signal decay, thus it is important that this gradient is reversed after the application of the RF pulse to revoke its effect on the signal decay (so called slice rewinding in this sense).

2.2.2. Phase- and Frequency Encoding

Once the slice is selected, the signal acquired from the slice does not include position encoding, so still a single peak is observed. The two remaining axis of the selected slice are the so called phase encoding and frequency encoding axis. After an RF pulse has flipped the spins, a gradient in the phase encoding direction is used to create a linear development in the Larmor frequency. This leads to a phase shift in the individual spins. When the phase encoding gradient is switched off, the generated phase shift persists in the spins.

A gradient on the frequency encoding axis changes the precession frequency of the protons in the sample. Protons under the influence of a larger gradient precess faster than protons influenced by a smaller frequency encoding gradient.

In most cases the phase encoding axis corresponds to the y-axis (up-down) of the slice and the frequency encoding axis corresponds to the x-axis (left-right direction). In the following, the terms y-axis and phase encoding axis are used as synonyms as well as the terms frequency encoding axis and x-axis are used equivalently.

2.3. Signal Echo Generation

The switching of gradients on the respective axes accelerates the signal decay and reduces the time available for signal acquisition. However, the effects introduced by additional gradients can be revoked and thus the signal can be recovered, with a slightly decreased strength due to T_1 and T_2 relaxation. This effect is called gradient echo generation and is schematically shown in figure 2.10. The first gradient which amplifies the signal decay is the so called dephasing gradient, while the echo generating gradient (up to the point until it reaches the same area A of the dephasing gradient) is the rephasing gradient.

A signal echo can also be generated by the application of a 180° pulse. This leads to a so called spin echo, in contrast to the gradient echo described before hand. More information on the generation of the spin echo can be found in e.g. [3]

2.4. k-Space Formalism

The effects of phase encoding and frequency encoding gradients are hard to imagine without the concept of k-space. K-space is a graphical 2D representation of the spins' frequency and phase within a measured slice. It is important to distinguish between k-space and image coordinates (and coordinate systems). The upper left corner of an image is NOT equivalent to the upper left corner of k-space.

2. Magnetic Resonance Imaging - The Very Basics

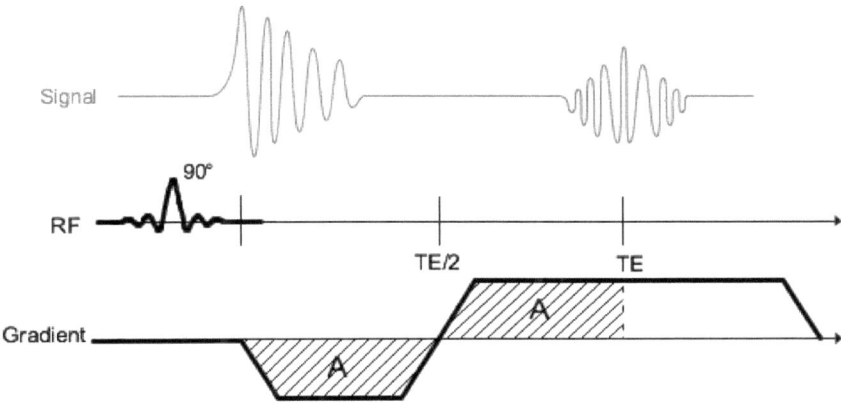

Figure 2.10.: *Signal echo generation by the application of gradients.*

Commonly, an image is described in x-y-coordinates, while k-space is in k_x-k_y-coordinates, where k_x is left-right direction and k_y is up-down direction. The mid-point of k-space has the coordinates (0,0). Every modification of the spins phase, or precession frequency reduces the signal, which can easily be observed in k-space. The center (which corresponds to no modification) is brighter than the outer region where the frequency and the phase of the spins are heavily modified by the applied gradients (figure 2.11).

The interesting thing about k-space is the easy access to the effect of image encoding gradients. In figure 2.12 the standard coordinate system for k-space is shown. After the RF pulse, all the spins have the same phase and precession frequency. This corresponds to the k-space origin (the center). A gradient in y-direction (phase encoding) changes the phase of the spins and moves to a different k_y position. A frequency encoding gradient changes the precession frequency and moves to a different k_x position. By subsequent playing of gradients along the frequency encoding and phase encoding axis a path through k-space (the so called trajectory) is defined.

The effect of a gradient in k-space is measured by the distance in k-space that has been covered during its on-time:

$$k_{x,y}(t) = \int_0^t \gamma h_{x,y}(t')dt' \qquad (2.3)$$

2. Magnetic Resonance Imaging - The Very Basics

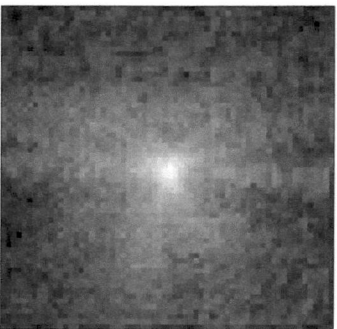

Figure 2.11.: *k-space of a brain image [1]; in the center the signal is brightest, diminishing to the outer regions*

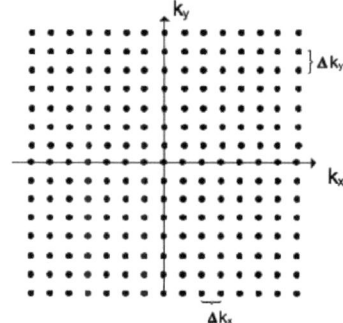

Figure 2.12.: *k-space coordinate system. The origin (0,0) is located in the center of the k-space*

with γ being the gyromagnetic ratio and $h(t)$ the gradient strength (or amplitude). A negative gradient amplitude corresponds to a movement downwards (or left, depending on the axis) and a positive gradient moves upwards (or right respectively). This correspondence is shown in figure 2.13. Along with the onset of a gradient is the onset of the analog to digital converter (ADC) which samples the signal. The number of points sampled during the onset of a gradient is defined by the sampling rate. In figure 2.13 the sampling positions are marked by dots on the gradients.

The digital sampling used in MRI splits the continuous signal into a discrete signal at different time points t_m. So for every sampled point the exact k-space position can be calculated using equation (2.3). If the k-space position at every point in time can be calculated, the imaging equation can be formulated in terms of the k-space coordinates:

$$s(k_x, k_y) = \iiint\limits_{x,y,z} \rho(x,y,z)\ sl(z)\ exp[-i2\pi(k_x x + k_y y)]\ dxdydz, \quad (2.4)$$

with $sl(z)$ being the slice excitation profile. From the imaging equation (2.4) it can be easily seen that the trajectory time course is encoded in the phase of the signal ($k_x x + k_y y$), whereas the magnitude represents the signal strength (spin density $\rho(x,y,z)$).

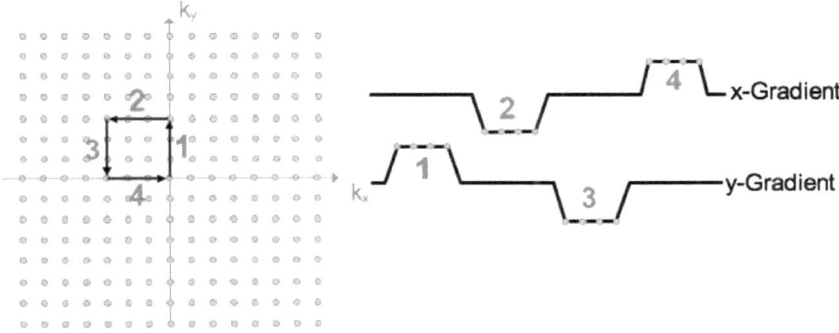

Figure 2.13.: *Effects of gradient switchings in k-space. Positive amplitude moves up (1) or right (4), negative amplitudes move down (3) or left (2), depending on the axis*

Bibliography

[1] E. M. Haacke, R. W. Brown, M. R. Thompson, and R. Venkatesan. *Magnetic Resonance Imaging - Physical Principles and Sequence Design*. Wiley-Liss, 1999.

[2] B. Blümich. *Essential NMR*. Springer Verlag, 2005. ISBN 3-540-23605-8.

[3] M. A. Bernstein, K. F. King, and X. J. Zhou. *Handbook of MRI Pulse Sequences*. Elsevier Academic Press, 2004. ISBN 0-12-092861-2.

3. Trajectory Design

In this chapter an overview of the background, and the actual design of the newly developed Hilbert-Moore trajectory is given. A survey of two existing standard gradient echo trajectories for MR image acquisition is presented in the first section 3.1. Afterwards a short introduction to space filling curves is given. Trajectory deviating effects are described in section 3.3. Details of the implementation and design decisions for the Hilbert-Moore trajectory are explained in section 3.4. In section 3.5 the validation of the trajectory is outlined. Finally, results of the implementation and the trajectory measurement are shown and evaluated in section 3.6.

3.1. Common Trajectories

The evolution in MR imaging goes along with the development of imaging trajectories. In the following section the FLASH (Fast Low Angle SHot) and the EPI (Echo Planar Imaging) trajectory are explained in more detail. Both trajectories are widely used and available on most MR imagers. EPI is today's gold standard for fMRI image acquisition and thus used as reference for the newly developed Hilbert-Moore sequence. EPI is based on FLASH, so in section 3.1.1 the FLASH trajectory is presented before in section 3.1.2 the EPI sequence is explained.

3.1.1. FLASH

All gradient echo sequences have in common that the signal echo is generated only by gradient reversal. In the following, the most basic gradient echo sequence, called FLASH (Fast Low Angle SHot) is presented in some detail.

The FLASH sequences traverses k-space in a line-wise fashion and a single line is acquired for each RF excitation. The basic concept of the gradient echo scheme can be easily understood using the k-space concept presented in 2.4. In figure 2.10 the effect

3. Trajectory Design

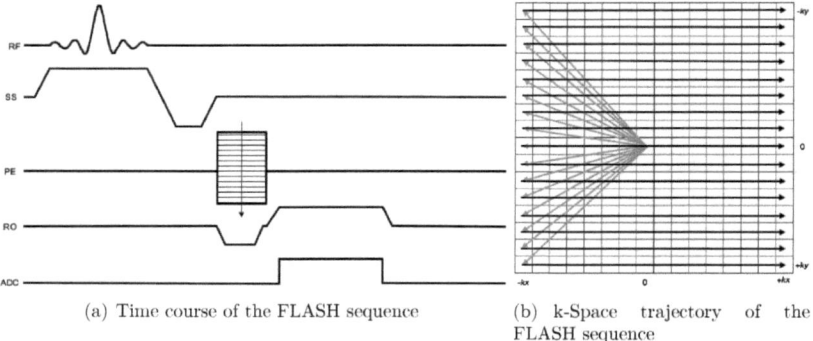

(a) Time course of the FLASH sequence

(b) k-Space trajectory of the FLASH sequence

Figure 3.1.: *Time course and k-space trajectory of the FLASH sequence. The dephasing and the phase encoding gradient move to the beginning of the line to be acquired. The readout gradient moves along the line. Data points are sampled during the plateau of the readout gradient*

of dephasing and rephasing gradients in k-space is shown. In FLASH, the dephasing gradient sets the actual sampling position from the k-space center to the beginning of one line, while the readout gradient encodes the different k-space positions along the line. Sampling occurs during the plateau of the readout gradient, during the on-time of the ADC (analog to digital converter). To acquire different lines of k-space, a phase-encoding (PE) table is used which encodes the actual line after the RF pulse has been played out. In the phase-encoding table the actual line to be imaged is tracked and the PE-gradient is adjusted accordingly. The complete time-course of the sequence and the resulting k-space trajectory is shown schematically in figure 3.1. The line-wise acquisition scheme with a new RF excitation for each line guarantees a good overall signal quality even for large resolutions. Image matrix sizes of 64×64 up to 512×512 pixels are easily possible with the FLASH sequence. The disadvantage of the FLASH sequence is the total image acquisition time. If e.g. a $90°$ pulse is used for excitation, the longitudinal magnetization has to be completely restored before the next line can be acquired, otherwise the signal strength will reduce considerably with each acquired line and thus reduce the overall image quality. Longer imaging time however increases the risk for motion artifacts and the discomfort for the subject inside the scanner. The use of smaller flip angles for the excitation allows for shorter repetition times (TR) and thus for faster acquisition. This reduces the overall signal strength but provides a consistent signal over the complete acquired k-space. To reduce the artifacts introduced by the shorter repetition times, so called spoiler or crusher gradients ([1]) are used to destroy remaining transversal magnetization.

3.1.2. Echo Planar Imaging

The Echo Planar Imaging sequence (EPI) is an imaging sequence based on the concept of the gradient echo sequence presented before. Instead of using multiple (one for every line as in FLASH) RF pulses for the acquisition of a slice, EPI uses one single RF pulse for each slice to be measured. Usually, a 90° RF pulse is applied for excitation and k-space is sampled with this single excitation (single shot). To retain the signal during sampling, a series of echoes (a so called echo-train) is generated by continuous dephasing and rephasing of the spins (figure 3.2). For each line to be measured, an echo is generated at the center of the line. The formation of the echo revokes the influence of the field gradients but T_2 relaxation is still effective, so the signal strength reduces for each echo. The k-space trajectory used in the EPI sequence is a modified zig-zag over the single k-space lines shown in figure 3.3.

In figure 3.4 the sequence time course is shown. It is the same idea as in the FLASH sequence. A dephasing gradient is applied (to set the actual sampling position to the beginning of the line in k-space), followed by a rephasing gradient (travel along the line). Applying a gradient with reversed polarity traverses back to the beginning of the line. Thus the second half of a gradient lobe serves as dephasing gradient for the next gradient lobe with opposite polarity. Also differently handled is the phase encoding. In the FLASH sequence, a phase encoding table is used that encodes the actual line to be acquired. For the EPI sequence, a single preparation gradient on the phase encoding axis is used that encodes the first line to be acquired. The next line to be acquired is then addressed by a short gradient blip after the current line has been sampled.

With modern gradient hardware, single shot EPI images can be acquired within a few tens of milliseconds, which is very convenient for applications like cardiac imaging, real-time imaging and other fields where fast imaging is necessary. For the fast sampling rates, a strong readout gradient with a high slewrate (the rate of rising the gradients amplitude) has to be used, which is very demanding for the gradient hardware.

The oscillating gradients and the single shot concept renders EPI susceptible to a

3. Trajectory Design

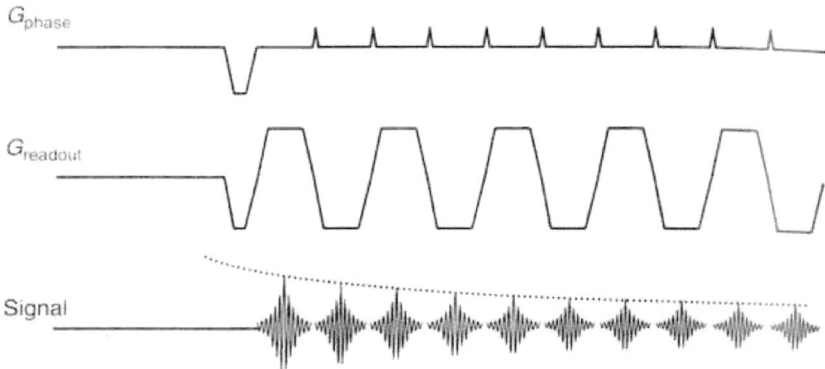

Figure 3.2.: *Echo train of the EPI sequence [1]. The second part of the previous gradient is used as the dephasing gradient to generate the echo. The overall signal strength, however, is decreasing nevertheless due to T_2 relaxation.*

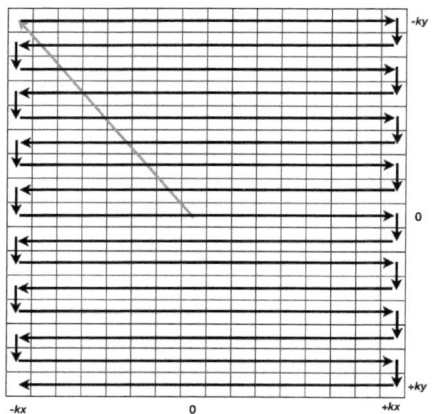

Figure 3.3.: *EPI trajectory represented in k-space*

3. Trajectory Design

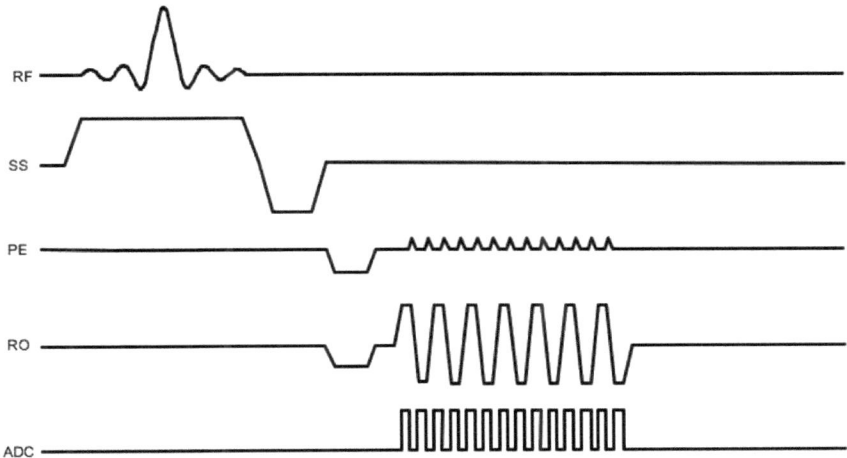

Figure 3.4.: *Time Course of a standard EPI sequence. The ADC sampling unit is switched on only during the plateau phases of the RO gradients.*

variety of artifacts. These artifacts are induced by several effects like off-resonance effects, B_0 field inhomogeneities and eddy currents. Especially eddy currents (section 3.3) are a big source of problems in EPI.

Another problem is the natural decay of the signal, that leads to severe image blurring. This can be overcome by sampling even faster so that the signal decay does not have a large influence. Another option is to switch to multishot techniques like interleaved or mosaic EPI ([1]).

The third major source of artifacts is the different polarity of the readout gradients. To correct for this alternating polarity, half of the rows have to be inverted, which leads to phase inconsistencies throughout k-space and thus to ghosting artifacts in the image.

Since EPI has already been proposed in 1977 by Sir Peter Mansfield, for most of these limitations a suitable correction algorithm has been developed until today, so that EPI is today's gold standard technique for several applications.

3.2. Space Filling Curves

The Hilbert-Moore sequence is based on the Hilbert-Moore space filling curve, so the concept of space filling curves is introduced in the following. After a general overview in section 3.2.1, the generation of Hilbert's space filling curve and Moore's modification of Hilbert's curve are presented in section 3.2.2. The only other application of space filling curves in MR is presented in section 3.2.3 and concludes the introduction to space filling curves.

3.2.1. History and Overview

Space filling curves are an interesting special case of fractal geometry. Mathematically spoken, a space filling curve is a continuous surjective mapping from an interval to a plane. It can neither be assigned the dimension of a curve (one dimensional) nor the dimension of a plane (two dimensional) but is somewhere in-between. In 1890, Peano proved the existence of such a curve. It was the answer to the question if a continuous surjective mapping from an interval into a plane can exist. After Peano presented his curve (figure 3.5), several others followed: Hilbert, Moore (both curves described in the following in more detail) and, among others, Sierpinski. The first graphical representation of a space filling curve was presented by Hilbert in 1891 (figure 3.6).

Space filling curves have quite a variety of possible applications, especially in the processing of multidimensional data sets. The standard representation of a two dimensional data set as a matrix is easily understandable but has a number of disadvantages. As shown in figure 3.7(a), the indices of neighboring points in a matrix can differ significantly, which leads not only to a certain calculation overhead but also to a fragmentation of the data in memory. Space filling curves, in contrast to the matrix representation, are mostly neighborhood preserving. This means that neighboring data points have similar indices, as can be seen in figure 3.7(b). This has advantages especially in the blockwise (e.g. parallel) processing of large data sets. The matrix order introduces a large overhead of memory operations to extract the block to be processed in advance of the actual processing. The data sorted along a space filling curve can be easily extracted and divided into separate blocks to be processed (figure 3.7(b)). More applications of space filling curves can be found in [2].

A complete introduction to space filling curves including a historic overview and sev-

3. Trajectory Design

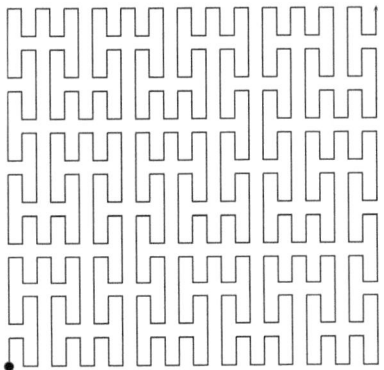

Figure 3.5.: *Peano's Space Filling Curve (Iteration 3)*

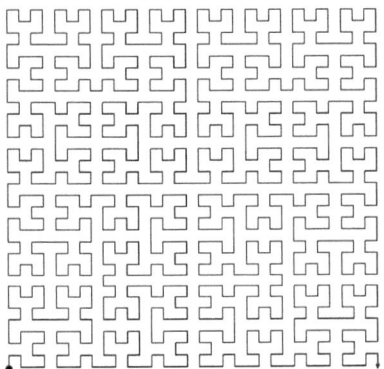

Figure 3.6.: *Hilbert's Space Filling Curve (Iteration 5)*

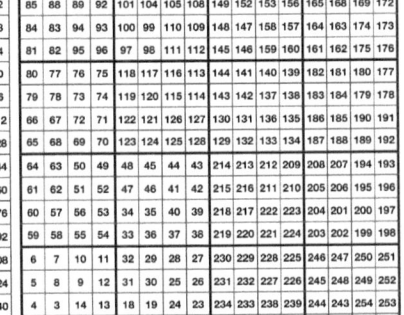

(a) Row Major Sorting

(b) Hilbert-Curve Sorting with possible block division for parallelization

Figure 3.7.: *Indices of a Matrix in (a) row major sorting and (b) Hilbert-Curve sorting*

eral properties of space filling curves can be found in [3]. In the following, the generation of Hilbert's space filling curves using grammars is outlined in more detail. Finally, a short excursion to cardiac imaging is done, before the (so far) only other application of space filling curves in magnetic resonance imaging is shortly explained.

3.2.2. Hilbert's Space Filling Curve

The grammar used to describe Hilbert's space filling curve consists of the nonterminal symbols $\{H, A, B, C\}$, the terminal symbols $\{\uparrow, \downarrow, \leftarrow, \rightarrow\}$, and H the start symbol. The following set of production rules defines the Hilbert curve:

$$
\begin{aligned}
H &\longleftarrow A \uparrow H \rightarrow H \downarrow B \\
A &\longleftarrow H \rightarrow A \uparrow A \leftarrow C \\
B &\longleftarrow C \leftarrow B \downarrow B \rightarrow H \\
C &\longleftarrow B \downarrow C \leftarrow C \uparrow A
\end{aligned}
$$

The graphic representation of this production rules, in combination with the basic patterns H, A, B, C is shown in figure 3.8. In figure 3.9 the first 3 iterations of Hilbert's space filling curve are presented. The main advantage of Hilbert's curve is the division of each (sub-)plane into $2^2 = 4$ subplanes. This allows for an easy integration into the matrix sizes needed for the efficient calculation of the fast Fourier transformation during image reconstruction. The total number of points covered by a Hilbert curve of iteration n is equal to 2^{2^n}. The sidelength of the square covered by this curve can be calculated by taking the square root of the number of points. In this work an iteration of 5 is used, which leads to 1024 points covering a 32x32 matrix, shown in figure 3.10.

Moore's Version Of Hilbert's Curve

Moore's version of Hilbert's curve changes the starting point of the curve. Regarding the curve in figure 3.10, it can be seen that the Hilbert curve starts at the lower left and ends at the lower right corner of the covered plane. The Hilbert-Moore curve shown in figure 3.11 emanates at the bottom line of the matrix, too, but in the middle column and ends at a directly adjacent point. By integration of an additional step, the curve can be easily closed and thus allows for a completely arbitrary starting point along the curve. This flexibility is exploited in the Hilbert-Moore sequence, where the choice of the start point determines the time to k-space center, the so called echo time TE.

3. Trajectory Design

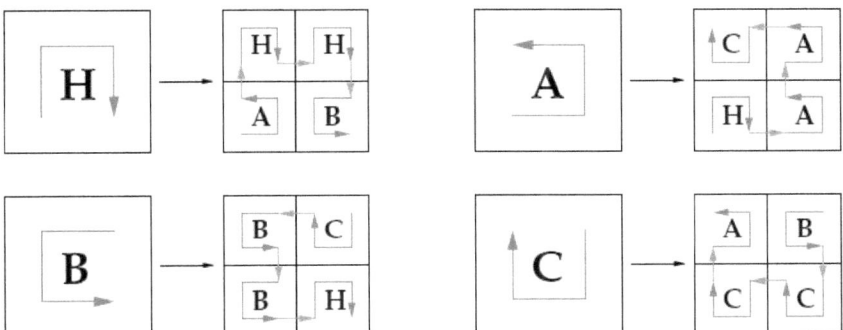

Figure 3.8.: *Patterns of the Hilbert Grammar [2] to recursively generate Hilbert's space filling curve*

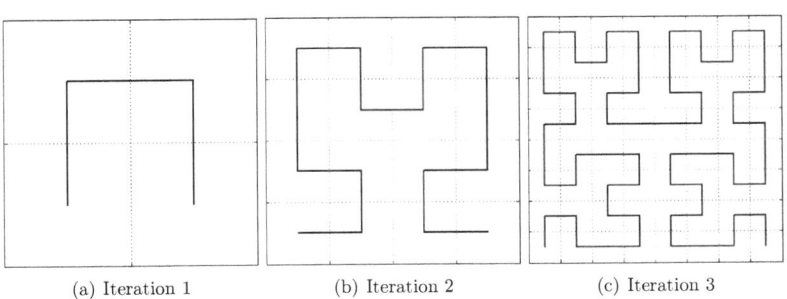

(a) Iteration 1 (b) Iteration 2 (c) Iteration 3

Figure 3.9.: *First three iterations of the Hilbert space filling curve. The replacement scheme described in the grammar can be clearly seen.*

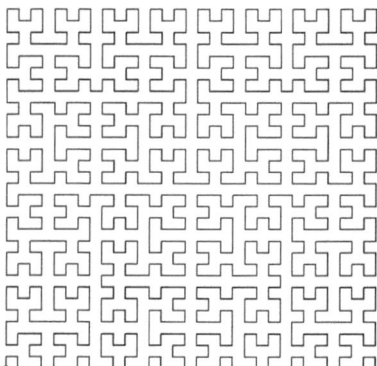
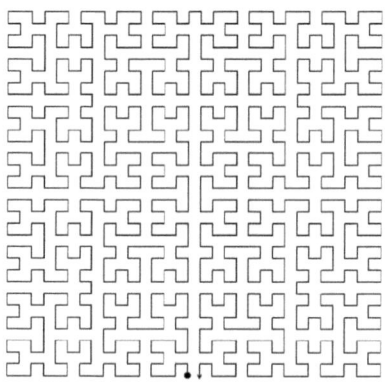

Figure 3.10.: *Iteration 5 of Hilbert's space filling curve, covering 1024 points in a 32x32 matrix.*

Figure 3.11.: *Iteration 5 of Hilbert-Moore space filling curve, covering 1024 points in a 32x32 matrix.*

3.2.3. Space Filling Curves In Magnetic Resonance

The only other known application of the Hilbert space filling curve has been proposed in 2007 [4] for cardiac imaging. Cardiac imaging with standard imaging sequences leads to severe artifacts and poor image quality due to the fast and complex motion of the heart. The standard technique is to monitor the cardiac cycle and acquire one k-space line at the same relative time after the heart-beat. This technique requires multiple heartbeats and multiple repetitions to acquire one slice. Several techniques to reduce imaging time have been proposed. The most common option distributes the acquisition of different k-space lines on distinct slices (one line per slice) over a complete cardiac cycle. The so called TRIADS (time resolved imaging with automatic data segmentation) scheme, which keeps track of the already acquired k_y-lines is shown in figure 3.12. The strategy on how to select the next k-space line has to be chosen carefully. Sudden jumps in k-space lead to eddy current artifacts (see section 3.3 for a description of eddy currents), which reduces image quality considerably.

Sigfriddson [4] extends the TRIADS scheme to take care of cardiac and respiratory gating. For each combination of cardiac and respiratory phase a separate time frame is acquired (figure 3.13) For each time frame, a progress counter is introduced which selects the next slice (k_z position) and line (k_y position) to be acquired. The neighborhood

3. Trajectory Design

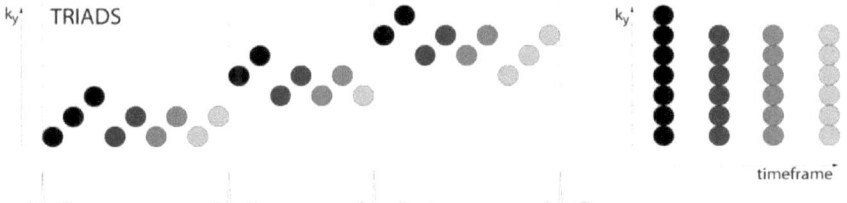

Figure 3.12.: *Time resolved imaging with automatic data segmentation (TRIADS) scheme for data acquisition in e.g. cardiac imaging. The TRIADS algorithm keeps track of the already acquired lines for each time frame and computes the next line to be acquired for a certain time frame (figure taken from [4])*

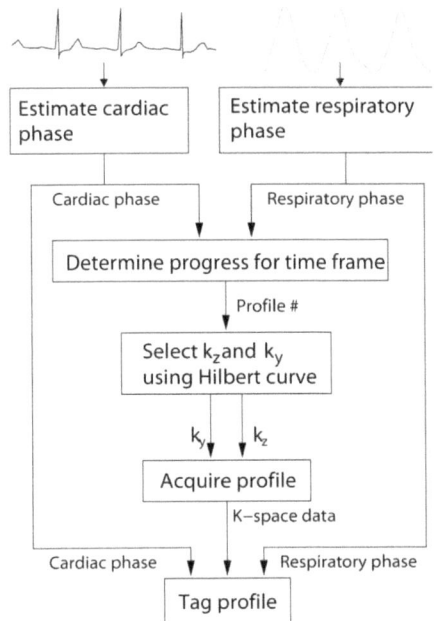

Figure 3.13.: *Cardiac and respiratory gated image acquisition proposed by Sigfridsson (figure taken from[4])*

3. Trajectory Design

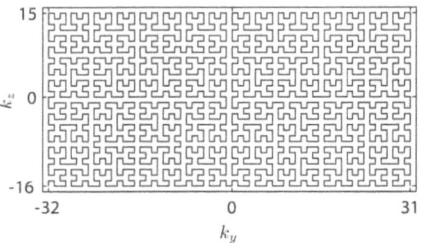

Figure 3.14.: *Selection order for the next slice (k_z) and line (k_y) position for the respiratory and cardiac gated image acquisition proposed by Sigfridsson. The acquisition starts in the lower left corner and ends in the lower right corner of the shown k_y-k_z-space (figure taken from [4])*

preservation of Hilbert's space filling curve is optimal in this sense. Sequential progress counters are mapped onto adjacent points in k_y-k_z space. The progress counter mapping function is shown in figure 3.14.

This approach sounds promising to overcome some of the limitations of cardiac imaging. Being proposed only recently, the outcome of this technique is not yet clear and has to be evaluated over the next years.

3.3. Trajectory Deviating Effects

The increase in gradient amplifier performance concerning slewrate and maximal amplitude as well as the use of higher field strength promote the building of trajectory deviating, local field inhomogeneities, mainly caused by eddy currents or gradient timing errors. Gradient timing errors are a technical problem and can be easily corrected by adopting the implementation to the actual timing needed for the gradient amplifier to switch the gradients properly. In contrast, eddy currents are a physical by-product of gradient switching. They depend on the gradient coil, the slewrate, and the gradient amplitude. In the following section, eddy currents are explained in greater detail. However the complete mathematical and physical background is beyond the scope of this thesis. A very comprehensive introduction and further references can be found in [1].

3. Trajectory Design

Eddy Currents

Faraday's law of induction describes the generation of a current in a coil when this coil is exposed to variations of magnetic flux. Following the trajectory in a pulse sequence leads necessarily, by switching of gradients, to variations in the magnetic flux. This changing flux induces currents in the structures of the MR imager as well as in the patient. In the patient, this generated current can lead to peripheral nerve stimulation [5]. In the conducting pathways of the MR imager, these currents (the so called eddy currents) induce a magnetic field which opposes the intended applied magnetic field that generated the eddy current (Lenz's law). Eddy currents build up during the time varying part of the gradient and decay within the constant part (during a plateau of the gradient waveform). The eddy currents of the rising and falling edge of a gradient have opposite signs and therefore partially cancel out after the waveform has been executed completely.

Time dependence of eddy currents can be modeled by a sum of decaying exponentials [6] with amplitude α_n and time constants τ_n. The constants α_n and τ_n depend on the coil hardware and have to be estimated empirically. The time constants can be divided into short term and long term time constants [1].

$$e(t) = H(t) \sum_n \alpha_n e^{-\frac{t}{\tau_n}} \text{ with } H(t) = \begin{cases} 1 & t \geq 0 \\ 0 & t < 0. \end{cases} \quad (3.1)$$

Adopting this model, the eddy current gradient $g_e(t)$ can be calculated

$$g(t) = -\frac{dG_{app}(t)}{dt} \otimes e(t), \quad (3.2)$$

where G_{app} is the applied gradient waveform and $\otimes$ denotes the convolution operation.

In the following, the effect of eddy currents on a gradient waveform is outlined. In general, the linear eddy currents are sufficient to describe the influence on the desired gradient waveform, so a single amplitude and time constant (α and τ) are used for the following calculations.

The applied gradient waveform G_{app} is characterized by the amplitude h and the rise time τ_{RT}:

$$G_{app}(t) = \frac{ht}{\tau_{RT}} \text{ with } 0 \leq t \leq r. \quad (3.3)$$

3. Trajectory Design

For the assumed single eddy current time constant, equation (3.2) evaluates to:

$$g(t) = -\frac{h}{\tau_{RT}}\alpha\tau(1 - e^{-\frac{t}{\tau}}). \tag{3.4}$$

The strength of the generated eddy current at the end of the rise time ($t = \tau_{RT}$) can be estimated using the previous equation. For a long term time constant $\tau \gg \tau_{RT}$, the term $e^{-\frac{\tau_{RT}}{\tau}}$ can be approximated by $1 + \frac{\tau_{RT}}{\tau}$ using the approximation rule $e^x \approx 1 + x$ for $x \ll 1$. Thus, the strength of the generated eddy current resolves to:

$$g_{rise}(t = \tau_{RT}) \approx -h\alpha. \tag{3.5}$$

For the falling edge of a waveform, the same considerations hold true but with the opposite sign of the amplitude:

$$g_{fall}(t = \tau_{RT}) \approx h\alpha. \tag{3.6}$$

So for long term time constants, the generated eddy current field depends only on the applied gradient amplitude h and is independent of the rise time, the slewrate, and the time constant. For a triangular waveform, with no constant gradient part where the eddy current gradient field decays, the resulting gradient waveform can then be described by:

$$\begin{aligned} G_{net}(t) &= G_{app,rise}(t) + g_{rise}(t) + G_{app,fall}(t) + g_{fall}(t) \\ &= G_{app,rise}(t) - h\alpha + G_{app,fall}(t) + h\alpha \\ &= G_{app,rise}(t) + G_{app,fall}(t). \end{aligned} \tag{3.7}$$

So the influence of eddy currents with long term time constants is negligible for a triangular gradient waveform.

For a short term time constant $\tau \ll \tau_{RT}$, the eddy current strength resolves to:

$$g(t) \approx -\frac{h\alpha\tau}{\tau_{RT}} \tag{3.8}$$

The applied gradient waveform then changes to:

$$G_{net}(t) = G_{app}(t) + g(t) \approx \frac{h(t - \alpha\tau)}{\tau_{RT}} = G_{app}(t - \alpha\tau), \tag{3.9}$$

3.4. Implementation Of The Hilbert-Moore Sequence

which cannot be distinguished from a time shift in the gradient amplifier and can thus be corrected by adjusting the timing of the gradient amplifier.

The following sections describe the considerations and design decisions to implement the Hilbert-Moore trajectory. In this work, the Hilbert-Moore sequence has been implemented for Siemens MRI-Scanners using the IDEA Software Version VB15. The IDEA programming environment is provided by Siemens and consists of the Microsoft Visual C++ Compiler, the CYGWIN environment, a cross compiler to generate the instruction file for the scanner, and several tools to simulate the interplay of the different components needed for a pulse sequence. The development of a pulse sequence is divided into two independent parts. The actual pulse sequence (that drives RF pulse, gradients and ADC) and a second part, the image reconstruction. As both components can be developed independently, the description of the implementation details is also separated. In the following, the implementation of the pulse sequence is outlined, while image reconstruction is described in chapter 4.

3.4.1. Design Considerations

The particularity of the Hilbert-Moore sequence is, in comparison to other sequences, the individual addressing of each sampling position. Especially in FLASH (section 3.1.1) and EPI (section 3.1.2), one complete k-space line is addressed and the sampling time of the single points is only controlled by the timing of the ADC. Depending on gradient amplitude (and thus on the speed used to travel k-space) the sampling time has to be adjusted so that the correct positions are sampled. The Hilbert-Moore gradient scheme is based on a completely different approach. Instead of long, trapezoidal shaped gradients, short triangular blips are used on both gradient axes to address k-space positions one after another following the order defined by the Hilbert-Moore space filling curve. This results in a feigned stochastic gradient switching with a fixed small gradient amplitude throughout the trajectory. The amplitude of the triangular blips depends on the field of view, the slewrate, and is constrained by the gradient raster time (GRT). In section 3.4.2 the calculation of the gradient blip amplitude is outlined in detail.

3. Trajectory Design

Gradient Shape

In the Siemens IDEA environment two predefined gradient shapes (trapezoidal and sinusoidal) can be used. In addition to these predefined shapes, an object *Arbitrary Shaped Ramps* exists that allows the sequence developer to define its own gradient shape. This object uses an array of numbers in the range of [-1,1] that define the outline of the gradient. The number of points that are used to define the shape of the arbitrary gradient is not limited. Along with the gradient shape, the maximum amplitude of the gradient is defined and a value of 1 inside the shape defining array corresponds to the maximum amplitude. In spite of its flexibility, some constraints have to be taken care of when using this method to define the gradients. First of all, the gradient amplifier does not allow for a continuous adjustment of the gradient shape but allows a change every $10\mu s$ (the gradient raster time, GRT) only. Furthermore, the gradient's slewrate has to be respected: The developer has to pay attention that no abrupt change of the gradient amplitude or direction occurs that can not be realized within the gradient raster time (GRT).

When implementing more complex trajectories like the Hilbert-Moore trajectory, two possibilities arise. Either the gradient shape is calculated during the preparation of the sequence using an analytical formula, or the gradient shape is pre-calculated and stored in a lookup table. In this work, the second method has been implemented. A lookup table for the gradient encoding and a second lookup table for the actual position in k-space have been build and hard-coded in the source-code. The starting position of the trajectory is (by default) set to the starting point of the Hilbert-Moore space filling curve (figure 3.11). An additional gradient step is encoded that closes the curve, so that the end point is equal to the starting point. The closed loop achieved by this additional step allows for an easy changing of the start point. It is ensured that sampling occurs on the complete trajectory and thus the k-space coverage is always the same, independent of the start point. The flexible choice of the starting point results in a flexible selection of the echo time. The echo time, being defined as the time to reach the k-space center, is directly dependent on the starting point of the Hilbert-Moore sequence. Choosing a starting point near but before the k-space center results in a very short echo time. A starting point on the trajectory near the k-space center but after the k-space center has already been sampled, results in a long echo time.

The gradient encoding table (Appendix A) does only consist of values {-1, 0, 1} depending on the direction of the next step along the curve. To respect the aforementioned constraints (GRT, slewrate), the value in the gradient encoding table is multiplied by a number of factors, depending on the total rise time for one gradient blip. This extension of the rise time is mandatory to stay within the slewrate limit. Details of the timing calculation can be found in section 3.4.2. If, for example, $40\mu s$ (4xGRT) are needed to achieve the necessary gradient moment for one blip, every step in the gradient encoding table is expanded by multiplication with the array {0.25, 0.50, 0.75, 1.00, 0.75, 0.50, 0.25, 0.00}. So the sequence {1,0,1} in the gradient encoding table would be expanded to the sequence {0.25, 0.50, 0.75, 1.00, 0.75, 0.50, 0.25, 0.00, 0.00, 0.00, 0.00, 0.00, 0.00, 0.00, 0.00, 0.00, 0.25, 0.50, 0.75, 1.00, 0.75, 0.50, 0.25, 0.00} in the gradient defining array.

Timing Considerations

Another objective to be taken into account is the total duration of the pulse sequence to cover k-space. In table 3.1 (page 37), the duration of one step in k-space for different field of view (FOV) sizes is outlined. For the standard image size used in functional MRI of 64×64 pixels, 64*64=4096, k-space points have to be covered. For the Hilbert-Moore sequence which addresses every k-space position individually this would result in 4096 steps (figure 3.15). Assuming a FOV of 250mm, every blip needs $40\mu s$ which leads to a total gradient switching time of about 160ms. Taking into account the preparation and slice selection gradients, about 200ms are needed per slice, with one RF excitation. Respecting the relaxation times in the range of 30 to 150ms, it can be seen that the signal strength has dropped considerably before the sampling has finished. To overcome this limitation, the number of sampling steps is reduced to 2048 and each blip extends over two k-space points instead of one (figure 3.15). The gaps introduced in the k-space matrix result in artifacts and are filled during image reconstruction using parallel imaging techniques. The description of how this is done can be found later on in chapter 4 where image reconstruction is explained in detail.

k-Space Center Sampling

The most important information for image quality is encoded in the k-space center region. For this reason, dense sampling of the k-space center region has been introduced in addition to the standard Hilbert-Moore trajectory. The k-space center region can be

3. Trajectory Design

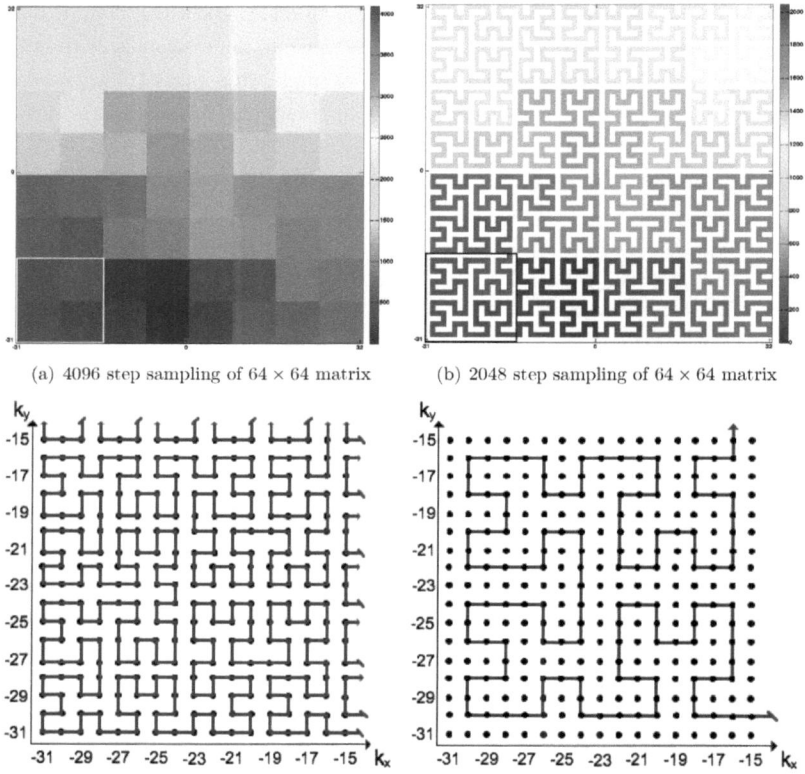

(a) 4096 step sampling of 64 × 64 matrix (b) 2048 step sampling of 64 × 64 matrix

(c) Lower left section of the 4096 step sampling (d) Lower left section of the 2048 step sampling

Figure 3.15.: *Comparison between the sampling of a 64 × 64 matrix with 4096 and 2048 steps. Figures (c) and (d) show the lower left bordered sections of figures (a) and (b) respectively. The dots in figure (c) and (d) mark positions in k-space. Sampled positions are covered by the trajectory. In figure (a) and (b), the color encodes the sampling order.*

3. Trajectory Design

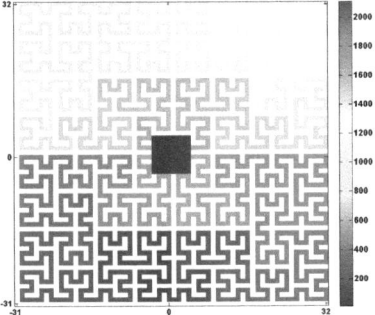

Figure 3.16.: *Preface variable density sampling, the additional sampled center region is sampled before the actual sequence trajectory is followed. Color encodes the actual sampling time point.*

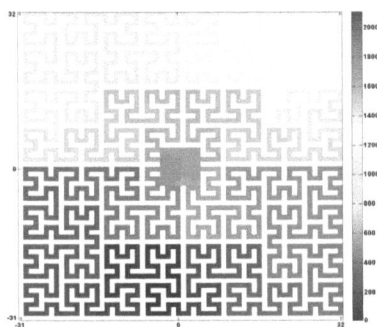

Figure 3.17.: *Inplace variable density sampling, the additional sampled center region is sampled when a certain point in the trajectory time course is reached. Color encodes the actual sampling time point.*

either sampled in advance or can be sampled at the time the trajectory enters the region covered by the variable density sampling. The resulting trajectories are shown in figure 3.16 and 3.17 respectively.

3.4.2. Gradient Amplitude Calculation

To follow the designed theoretical trajectory, the exact sampling position of k-space points is very important. Even if the trajectory can be corrected for small deviations using interpolation schemes like Gridding [7], the exact timing and gradient setting for the trajectory to be followed is crucial for image quality. For the Hilbert-Moore gradient scheme both parameters (gradient amplitude and duration) can be calculated easily once the Delta-Moment (the gradient strength needed to move from one k-space position to the adjacent one) is known. In the following, the theoretical equation framework is given to calculate a triangle blip of minimal duration to move one step in k-space. The developed formulas are applied to different FOVs in section 3.6.1.

3. Trajectory Design

Theoretical Framework

Let Δ be the gradient moment needed to move the trajectory from one k-space grid position to the directly adjacent one. For all gradient shapes, the zeroth order moment (which corresponds to Δ) is the integral of the gradient waveform. Regarding a triangular waveform, the integral corresponds to the area of the triangle and can be calculated by

$$A = \frac{g \cdot h}{2} \tag{3.10}$$

where h is the triangle height and g the length of the triangle base. Carried on to gradients, g equals the time during which the gradient is different from zero, h is the peak amplitude of the gradient, and A corresponds to Δ.

For the Hilbert-Moore gradient waveform with its high number of gradient switchings, it is important to keep the time needed for one gradient step as short as possible. Therefore the aim is therefore to find the minimal time needed for the waveform to achieve a certain Δ. For a triangular waveform the minimal amount of time equals two times the risetime. The risetime τ_{RT} is defined to be the ratio of amplitude (h) and slewrate (SR). Thus, the length of the basis g (the total gradient on-time) can be expressed as:

$$g = 2 \cdot \tau_{RT} = 2 \cdot \frac{h}{SR}. \tag{3.11}$$

Inserting equation (3.11) into equation (3.10), this can be solved for h:

$$h = \pm\sqrt{SR \cdot \Delta} \tag{3.12}$$

Once the amplitude has been calculated using equation (3.12), the gradient on-time g can be calculated using equation (3.11). After the exact time τ_{RT} needed to achieve the amplitude h has been evaluated, the gradient raster time has to be taken into account, and the time τ_{RT} has to be rounded to the next multiple of 10, yielding τ_{GRT}. This new timing parameter is now inserted into equation (3.10) and the final amplitude h' can be calculated. The necessary Delta-Moment Δ, the minimum risetime and the resulting maximal slewrate can be acquired and caluclated using methods provided by the IDEA framework.

3. Trajectory Design

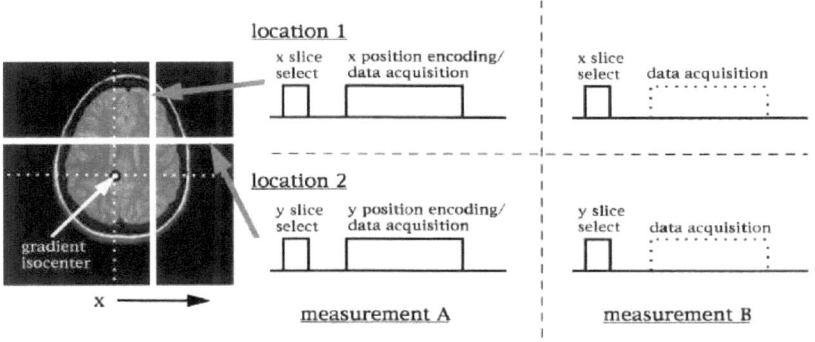

Figure 3.18.: *Scheme of Duyn Trajectory Measurement [8]*

3.5. Trajectory Verification

Once the trajectory has been designed and implemented, it can be executed on the scanner. Unfortunately, a variety of physical effects and hardware imperfections exist that can disturb the theoretical designed course of the trajectory. This leads to the necessity to measure the actual trajectory and, in case of serious deviations, correct for these inconsistencies. The type of artifacts introduced by trajectory deviations depends on the trajectory itself, e.g. in the EPI sequence a k-space shift causes ghosting artifacts. Other possible effects of trajectory deviations are compression, shearing or a displacement of the object in the final image.

Duyn Trajectory Measurement

The algorithm proposed by Duyn [8] is very simple and can easily be integrated into a standard MR measurement. It can be executed with the object to be measured being present inside the scanner and thus excludes the inconsistencies coming from a change of the object to be measured. Each direction of spatial encoding is measured separately by two scans. The slice selection gradient is switched to the axis of spatial encoding that is to be measured, and gradients on other axes are switched off. Two measurements for each encoding axis are to be done. The first measurement is executed with the slice selection gradient and the encoding gradient being active. For the second measurement, the encoding gradient is switched off, and only the slice selection gradient on the respective axis is played out. In figure 3.18 this is exemplarily shown for x- and y-encoding axis. Data acquisition is switched on as normal.

The switching of the slice selection gradient to a gradient encoding axis excites a slice with a certain thickness along this axis and complete coverage of the other two encoding dimensions. As no other gradient is executed, the phase of the acquired signal consists only of the encoding gradient for the respective axis and the influence of the slice selection gradient on this axis (figure 3.18, measurement A).

For the second measurement B (figure 3.18), with the encoding gradient switched off, the phase of the acquired signal consists only of the influence of the slice selection gradient:

To filter out disturbing effects introduced by the slice selection gradient, the difference of the phase of the two signals is taken. This phase difference can be expressed as:

$$\Delta\phi_{x,y}(t) = \int_0^t \gamma \cdot G_{x,y}(t) \cdot D_{x,y} \cdot dt = D_{x,y} \cdot k_{x,y}(t), \qquad (3.13)$$

where $D_{x,y}$ is the distance between the gradient iso-center and the selected slice on the respective axis. The gradient time course can be calculated by normalization of equation (3.13) to the distance $D_{x,y}$. Best results are achieved if the slice thickness is small compared to the distance $D_{x,y}$.

3.6. Results

This section lists the implementation results for the Hilbert-Moore sequence. Firstly, the calculation of the gradient amplitudes and the intended trajectory with the associated gradient scheme is shown. Afterwards, the complete sequence time course including RF pulse, slice selection gradient and ADC readouts is illustrated. After an analysis of the possible artifacts that can appear when the trajectory deviates from its ideal course, the results from the trajectory measurements are presented.

3.6.1. Gradient Amplitudes

In table 3.1 the calculated amplitude h and risetime τ_{RT}, as well as the final amplitude h' (with respect to the gradient raster time) are shown for different FOV.

3. Trajectory Design

Table 3.1.: *Amplitude h' and blip risetime τ_{RT} for the Siemens TRIO 3T system and the Siemens Avanto 1,5T system with a maximal slewrate of $170\ mT/(m\cdot ms)$*

FOV [mm]	Δ [$mT\cdot\mu s/m$]	h [mT/m]	$\tau_{\mathbf{RT}}$ [μs]	$\tau_{\mathbf{GRT}}$ [μs]	h' [mT/m]
194	121,07	6,41	37,73	40	6,05
200	117,43	6,32	37,16	40	5,87
250	93,95	5,65	33,23	40	4,69
300	78,29	5,16	30,34	40	3,91
306	76,75	5,10	30,04	40	3,83
313	75,04	5,05	29,70	30	5,00
400	58,71	4,46	26,27	30	3,91
500	46,97	3,99	23,50	30	3,13

The resulting gradient scheme with the small amplitude blips on the x- and y-axis is shown in figure 3.19. Some sampling time points are marked exemplarily for the normal sampling scheme and the densely sampled k-space center.

3.6.2. Sequence Time Course

The exact sequence time course depends on a variety of parameters. Schematically, the Hilbert-Moore sequence time course can be divided into four parts:

1. RF pulse and slice selection gradients,

2. Preparation gradients to set a certain starting point,

3. Trajectory gradients,

4. Variable density gradients.

Step 4, the VD sampling step, can be executed at two different time points. Figure 3.20 shows the difference in the two options: Figure 3.20(a) shows the sequence time course with the variable density acquisition before the execution of the complete sequence (Preface), i.e. the VD sampling is inserted inbetween step 1 and 2. It is clear that additional preparation gradients are needed but the complete k-space is sampled in one long readout. In figure 3.20(b) the variable density sampling scheme is inserted inside (Inplace) the k-space spanning trajectory. This time only one pair of preparation gradients is needed but the readout is split into three parts, which have to be merged before the reconstruction.

3. Trajectory Design

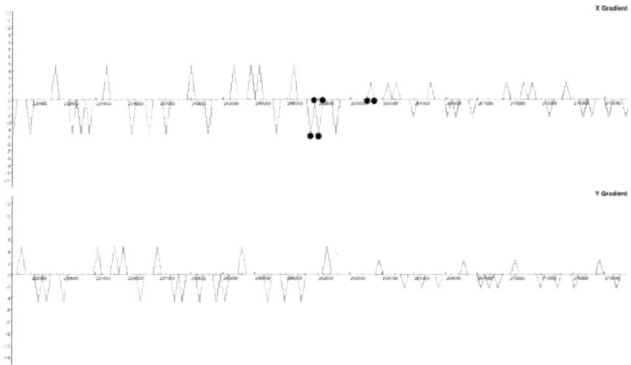

Figure 3.19.: *Gradient blips and amplitudes of the Hilbert-Moore trajectory. Smaller blips correspond to the densely sampled center region. Some exemplary sampling time points are marked.*

The echo time of the sequence depends on the starting point in k-space. The Hilbert-Moore sequence samples k-space in a circular fashion, which means that the end-point of the trajectory time course equals the start-point. Depending on the position in k-space where the sequence starts, the time to the k-space center position is different, relying on the number of steps needed to reach k-space center.

3.6.3. Trajectory Deviation Simulation

The artifacts introduced by trajectory deviation have been investigated by simulation. The imaging equation (2.4) reveals that a deviation from the trajectory can be expressed by a phase shift in the signal. In the simulation this behavior is implemented by adding a random value ϕ_d with $-\pi \leq \phi_d \leq \pi$ to the phase of the signal simulated under the assumption of a perfect trajectory. The amount of k-space points can be stated by the user before the simulation begins. In figure 3.21 the images of a simulation for an increasing number of phase errors is shown. It can be seen that the Hilbert-Moore sequence is quite robust with regard to phase errors: even with most of the trajectory data being distorted, the object to be imaged is still visible. Another interesting point is the effect of the phase errors. In contrast to EPI where shifts in k-space lead to clearly visible ghosting artifacts, k-space shifts in the Hilbert-Moore sequence increase the background

3. Trajectory Design

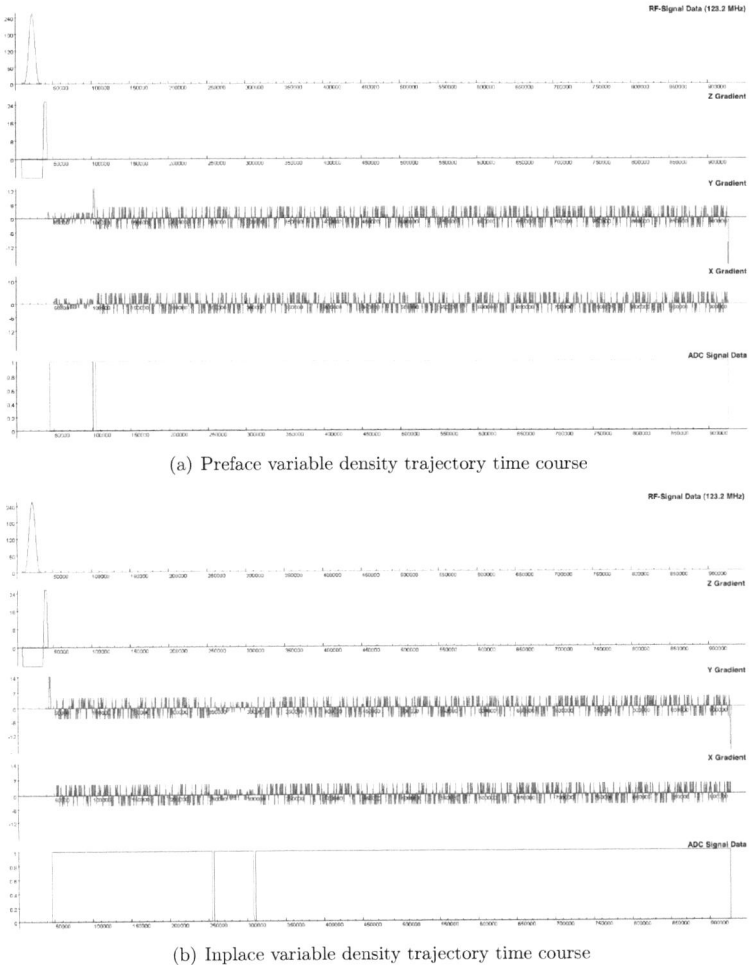

(a) Preface variable density trajectory time course

(b) Inplace variable density trajectory time course

Figure 3.20.: *Variable density time course for the Hilbert-Moore sequence. In (a), the preface variable density time course, the sampling of the center, occurs before the actual sampling of the trajectory and thus only two ADC events are needed. In (b), three ADC are needed, because of the split of the trajectory into a preVD and a postVD part. The high gradient peaks correspond to the preparation gradients needed to set the desired startpoint (in this case (0,-30)). The figures have been generated with the sequence simulation toolkit POET provided with the IDEA framework*

3. Trajectory Design

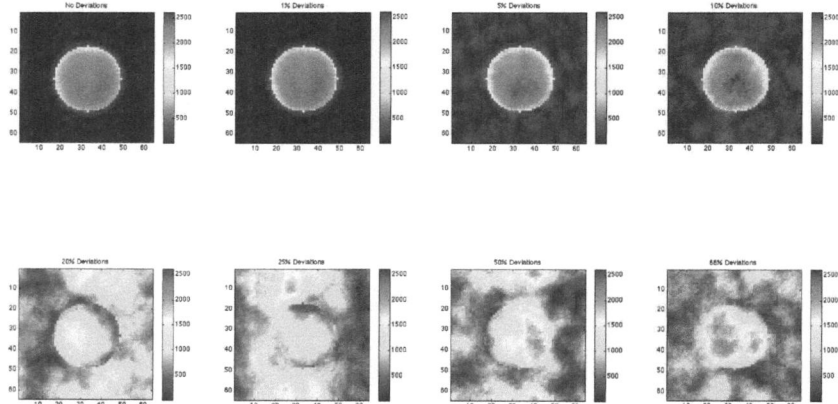

Figure 3.21.: *Different amounts of phase errors introduced into the Hilbert-Moore sequence data before the reconstruction takes place.*

noise. This is also due to ghosting artifacts but the doubled undersampling inherent in the Hilbert-Moore sequence distributes the ghosting artifacts over the image instead of focussing to fixed positions like in EPI.

3.6.4. Trajectory Measurement

In figure 3.22 the measured trajectory is overlaid on the designed trajectory. The very good correspondence between the designed and the measured trajectory confirm the calculated theoretical results. The Hilbert-Moore trajectory, is due to its triangular gradient waveform hardly susceptible to distortions of the trajectory introduced by eddy currents as shown in section 3.3.

The outliers seen in the upper left corner of figure 3.22 are at maximum a shift of about one k-space step for the x-direction. The mean absolute difference between the measured and the designed trajectory is about 0.05 for k_x-direction and about 0.04 for the k_y-direction. Δk, the distance between two adjacent points in k-space is about 0.1 for k_x and k_y direction.

The Hilbert-Moore sequence follows the designed trajectory quite accurately and in addition is self-regulatory: the inconsistencies in the upper left corner in figure 3.22 are

3. Trajectory Design

Figure 3.22.: *Overlay of measured (stippled red) and designed (blue) trajectory*

compensated by the following gradients and are dissolved when the trajectory reaches the center portion of k-space and its end point.

3.7. Discussion

The design of the Hilbert-Moore sequence was relatively straight forward. Starting from Hilbert's space filling curve on a 32×32 k-space matrix to the final 64×64 undersampled Hilbert-Moore trajectory, a number of constraints had to be respected. Due to the high number of gradient switchings, the Hilbert-Moore sequence is quite demanding for the scanner hardware and one of the main counter-arguments has been that the scanner is not capable of playing such a gradient scheme in a reasonable amount of time. With the introduction of the twofold undersampling the fMRI standard 64×64 k-space matrix can be sampled in a practically relevant amount of time with an appropriate image quality.

It has furthermore been shown that eddy currents (the second most objection against the Hilbert-Moore sequence) do not introduce errors into the Hilbert-Moore sequence. Due to the triangular sampling scheme, the build up of an eddy current is followed by the build up of a similar eddy current in the opposite direction. Thus, it can be said that the build up of an eddy current is directly followed by its dismantling.

3. Trajectory Design

The time discontinuity introduced in the sampling of adjacent data points along the middle axis of the image remains an open question. In the following section on image reconstruction, it is evaluated, which influence this time gap provides on the image quality.

Another objective is Peripheral Nerve Stimulation (PNS). The time varying magnetic fields generated by the gradients give rise to electric fields that may stimulate nerves or muscles in the subject lying inside the scanner. This is a major safety concern and a threshold for the variation of the magnetic fields (expressed in $\frac{dB}{dt}$) has been defined. The threshold value of the common stimulation model can be calculated using the formula ([5]):

$$\frac{dB}{dt} = \frac{54T}{s}(1 + \frac{138\mu s}{pulseduration[\mu s]}) \qquad (3.14)$$

Inserting the duration of a gradient pulse for the Hilbert-Moore sequence ($40\mu s$), a threshold value of 240T/s has to be achieved before PNS may occur. As an approved medical device, the scanner checks automatically if this threshold is exceeded for the actual sequence or not and displays a warning message or does not allow to execute the sequence. The actual stimulation value of the sequence being played out can also be investigated, and for the Hilbert-Moore sequence the values are at about ~75% of the maximum value allowed.

In conclusion it can be said, that the Hilbert-Moore sequence is a robust sequence, even with its high demand to the gradient hardware. Despite the high number of gradient switchings, the Hilbert-Moore sequence is well within the safety limits defined by national standards. The new design with the individual addressing of the k-space points suggests a variety of improvements like correction of the signal decay. For these corrections, however, the influence of each single spin ensemble has to be calculated for each individual point, which would lead to a large computational overhead.

Bibliography

[1] M. A. Bernstein, K. F. King, and X. J. Zhou. *Handbook of MRI Pulse Sequences.* Elsevier Academic Press, 2004. ISBN 0-12-092861-2.

[2] M. Bader. *Raumfüllende Kurven.* Technische Universität München, 2004.

[3] H. Sagan. *Space-Filling Curves.* Springer Verlag, 1994.

[4] A. Sigfridsson, J. P. E. Kvitting, H. Knutsson, and L. Wigström. Five-dimensional MRI incorporating simultaneous resolution of cardiac and respiratory phases for volumetric imaging. *Journal of Magnetic Resonance Imaging*, 25:113–121, 2007.

[5] D. J. Schaefer, J. D. Bourland, and J. A. Nyenhuis. Review of patient safety in time-varying gradient fields. *Journal of Magnetic Resonance Imaging*, 12(1):20–29, 2000.

[6] P. Jehenson, M. Westphal, and N. Schuff. Analytical method for the compensation of eddy-current effects induced by pulsed magnetic field gradients in NMR systems. *Journal of Magnetic Resonance*, 90:264–278, 1990.

[7] J. I. Jackson, C. H. Meyer, D. G. Nishimura, and A. Macovski. Selection of a convolution function for fourier inversion using gridding [computerised tomography application]. *IEEE Transactions on Medical Imaging*, 10(3):473–478, 1991.

[8] J. H. Duyn, Y. Yang, J. A. Frank, and J. W. van der Veen. Simple correction method for k-space trajectory deviations in MRI. *Journal of Magnetic Resonance*, 132:150–153, 1998.

4. Image Reconstruction

Usually, an MR image is reconstructed by application of a Fourier transformation to the acquired frequency and phase encoded signal. For the Hilbert-Moore sequence with the twofold undersampling, it is not as easy. A special reconstruction algorithm had to be developed that fills the gaps in k-space before the Fourier Transformation is applied. In this chapter the image reconstruction algorithm for the Hilbert-Moore sequence is presented. Firstly, a short introduction to parallel imaging, SMASH, PARS, GRAPPA, and the MCMLI algorithm is given in section 4.1. Afterwards the design and implementation of the Hilbert-Moore reconstruction algorithm is explained in 4.2. Images reconstructed from simulation and scanner data finish this chapter along with the discussion of the results.

4.1. Parallel Imaging

Parallel imaging is the general notion for imaging techniques that use multiple coils (in parallel) to acquire the signal. When it came up, the intention of parallel imaging has been to increase the signal-to-noise-ratio by calculating the mean value of the multiple acquisitions. Soon after the establishment of multiple receiver coils, the first approaches to reduce scan time by leaving out k-space lines and reconstruct the missing information using the multiple coil data have been presented. The introduction of gaps into the k-space matrix leads to the necessity to either fill these gaps in k-space or to unwrap the aliased image generated from the incomplete k-space matrix. The most popular approaches are SMASH (Simultaneous Acquisition of Spatial Harmonics) [1] and SENSE (Sensitivity Encoding for fast MRI) [2]. SMASH is a k-space based technique and reconstructs missing pixels in k-space. It is the predecessor of GRAPPA (Generalized Autocalibrating Partially Parallel Acquisitions) [3] and will be described in more detail in section 4.1.1. SENSE is an image space based technique and unfolds the overlapping pixels introduced by the reconstruction with gaps in k-space present. Both techniques have advantages in different fields of application so it is impossible to say which technique is superior. In this work, a k-space based technique seemed more promising due to the regular, self similar k-space trajectory of the Hilbert-Moore sequence.

In the following, SMASH (4.1.1) is presented before its enhancement PARS (Parallel Imaging with Adaptive Radius in k-Space) [4, 5] (4.1.2), a sliding window reconstruction technique, is described. The autocalibrating enhancement for SMASH called GRAPPA (4.1.3) is presented afterwards. This section on parallel imaging is concluded with a short description of the MCMLI (Multi-Column-Multi-LIne) [6] (4.1.4) enhancement of the GRAPPA algorithm.

4.1.1. SMASH

SMASH, SiMultaneous Acquisition of Spatial Harmonics [1], was the first imaging technique that used multiple receive coils to speed up the acquisition process of an MR image. More precisely, the linear combination of the coil sensitivity weighted data is used to synthesize lines in k-space which can then be left out during the acquisition. Thus a reduced amount of data is acquired, which leads to a reduction in imaging time.

A receive coil does not have a uniform sensitivity, instead a monotonic fall off of the sensitivity can be observed with increasing distance from the coil. This behavior has to be included into the imaging equation by an additional term $C(x,y)$ which represents the coil sensitivity:

$$S(k_x, k_y) = \int \int C(x,y) \rho(x,y) exp(-i(k_x x + k_y y)) dx dy. \tag{4.1}$$

Assuming that multiple coils, with distinct but overlapping coil sensitivities $C_l(x,y)$ (where l represents the coil index) can be linearly combined using weights w_l, so that the composite sensitivity yields the form of a complex exponential of the k-space distance Δk_y (with m being an integer):

$$C^{comp}(x,y) = \sum_l w_l C_l(x,y) = exp(im\Delta k_y y). \tag{4.2}$$

The combined MR signal of these coils is shifted in k-space by exactly the same amount

$m\Delta k_y$:

$$S(k_x, k_y) = \int\int C^{comp}(x,y)\rho(x,y)exp(-i(k_x x + k_y y))dxdy \qquad (4.3)$$
$$= \int\int \rho(x,y)exp(-i(k_x x + (k_y - m\Delta k_y)y))dxdy$$
$$= FFT[\rho(k_x, k_y + m\Delta k_y)].$$

So for known coil sensitivities, nearly any k-space point can be calculated out of another one if the distance in k-space between the two points can be expressed by a spatial harmonic. For omitting every second line during acquisition, only the direct neighbours ($m = \pm 1$) are used for the reconstruction(see also figure 4.1):

$$S(k_x, k_y) = \int\int \rho(x,y)exp(-i(k_x x + k_y y))dxdy \qquad (4.4)$$
$$= \int\int \rho(x,y)exp(-i(k_x x + (k_y - m\Delta k_y + m\Delta k_y)y))dxdy$$
$$= \int\int C^{comp}(x,y)\rho(x,y)exp(-i(k_x x + (k_y - m\Delta k_y)y))dxdy$$
$$= \int\int \sum_l w_l C_l(x,y)\rho(x,y)expt(-i(k_x x + (k_y + m\Delta k_y)))dxdy$$
$$= \sum_l w_l \int\int C_l(x,y)\rho(x,y)exp(-i(k_x x + (k_y + m\Delta k_y)))dxdy$$
$$= \sum_l w_l S_l(k_x, k_y + m\Delta k_y).$$

4.1.2. PARS

Parallel Imaging with Adaptive Radius in k-Space (PARS, [4, 5]) is a k-space based reconstruction scheme for parallel imaging that uses a k-space locality criterion to select the points used to reconstruct a missing point. Based on the fact that nearby points are acquired with (nearly) the same coil sensitivity, only points within a certain radius around the missing point are used for the reconstruction (figure 4.1).

The data reconstruction equation of PARS involves additional summations to cover the points inside the radius (where n is an integer expressing neighboring column index):

$$S(k_x, k_y) = \sum_l \sum_n \sum_m w_{l,n,m} S_l(k_x + n\Delta k_x, k_y + m\Delta k_y). \qquad (4.5)$$

In comparison to the SMASH algorithm, not a single (well defined) line is used to recon-

4. Image Reconstruction

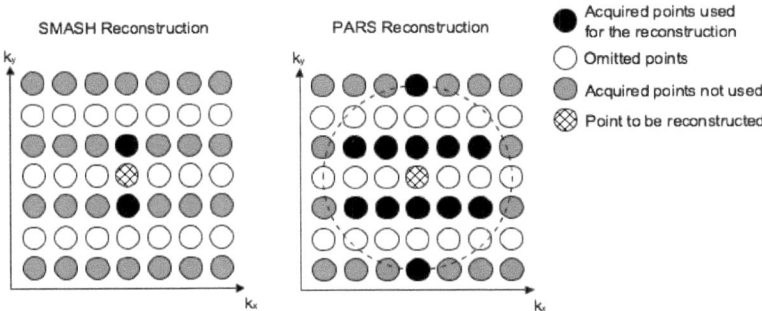

Figure 4.1.: *Comparison of the SMASH and the PARS reconstruction scheme. In SMASH only the direct neighbors are used for the reconstruction. In PARS a circle around the point to be reconstructed is used to select the points used for the reconstruction. The data-sets for a single coil are shown for reasons of simplicity.*

struct a missing point; but for each missing point, the source points for the reconstruction are selected dynamically.

4.1.3. GRAPPA

The major drawback of SMASH and PARS is the separate acquisition of the coil sensitivity profiles. This additional measurement renders the sensitivity estimation imprecisely and could result in serious artifacts. GRAPPA [3] extends the SMASH algorithm with an autocalibration technique so that no separate acquisition of the coil sensitivities is necessary.

In GRAPPA several autocalibration lines are acquired near the center of k-space (figure 4.2). These autocalibration lines (ACS) are included into the image to improve image quality, and are also used to estimate the weights w_l needed for the combination of the signals, shown in equation (4.4). To improve image quality, GRAPPA additionally does not generate a single overall image (as SMASH does) but reconstructs individual coil images which are then combined using the sum of squares.

The complex combination weights in equation (4.4) can be found by solving a linear system if the point on the left side of the equation (the point to be reconstructed) and the points on the right side of the equation (the source points) are known. The GRAPPA

4. Image Reconstruction

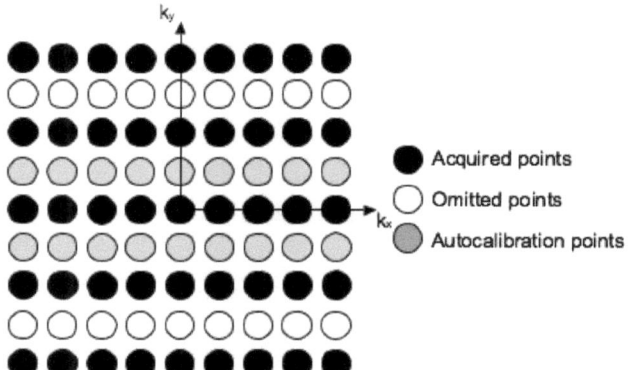

Figure 4.2.: *Variable density autocalibrating acquisition scheme for GRAPPA. The black points mark normally acquired points. The white points mark points left out during acquisition and the gray points mark the additionally acquired variable density points used for the autocalibration.*

algorithm uses the additionally acquired autocalibration data to estimate the weights used to reconstruct the image in the coil u from the other coils in this way:

$$S_u^{ACS}(k_x, k_y) = \sum_l w_{lu} S_l(k_x, k_y - m\Delta k_y). \qquad (4.6)$$

Written in matrix formulation, the calculation of the weights is straightforward:

$$S^{ACS} \equiv R = WS \qquad (4.7)$$
$$RS^{-1} = W.$$

The difficulty is that the matrix S cannot be inverted directly (it is usually not a quadratic matrix) but the Moore-Penrose pseudo-inverse has to be used. The calculated weights are thus not the exact solution but an approximation to the real weights which cannot be calculated without a separate coil sensitivity acquisition. In figure 4.3 the GRAPPA weight calculation is depicted schematically. The weighting matrix W is of size LxL where L is the total number of coils used. Each matrix element $[w]_{lu}$ is the combination weight of the coil sensitivity of the coil l to form the respective spatial

4. Image Reconstruction

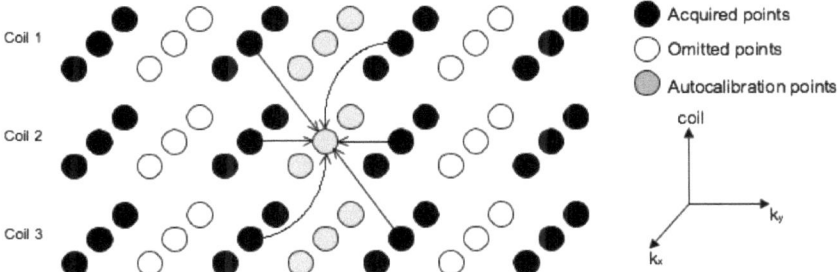

Figure 4.3.: *GRAPPA weight calculation for a single coil (coil 2). All points used later on for the reconstruction are fitted to the respective autocalibration point, and the weights are calculated by solving the resulting linear system. Only points with the same k_x coordinate are used.*

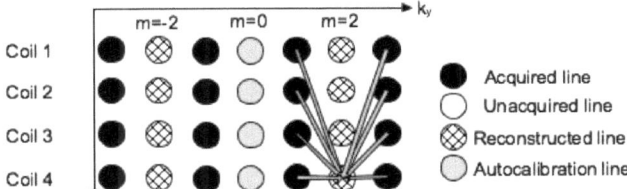

Figure 4.4.: *GRAPPA reconstruction scheme; the calculated weights (figure 4.3) from the autocalibration data are used to reconstruct missing data lines over the complete k-space using same neighborhood relations.*

harmonic for the coil u.

The calculated weights are now used to reconstruct missing lines overall the complete k-space matrix and separate images for each coil are calculated. Finally, the separate coil images are combined into a single image using the sum of squares algorithm.

The GRAPPA algorithm is not applicable to the Hilbert-Moore sequence in its original form. Differences in the signal strength for outer k-space regions are respected inherently in the calculation of the weights. For each k_x-position a separate weight w_{lu} is calculated. For the Hilbert-Moore sequence with its twofold undersampling, it is impossible to calculate a weight for every k_x position of k-space. This restriction to fully sampled lines and reconstruction of missing phase-encoding lines only renders the GRAPPA al-

4. Image Reconstruction

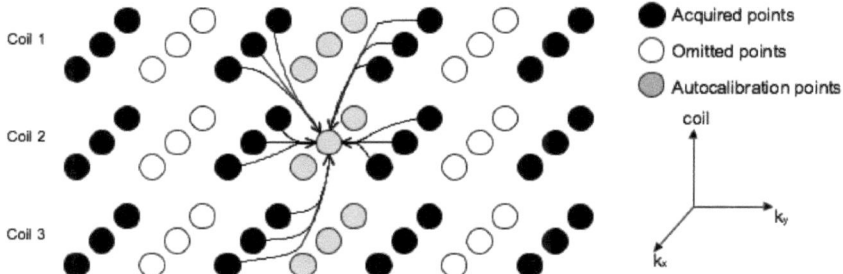

Figure 4.5.: *MCMLI weight calculation for a single coil (coil 2). All points used later on for the reconstruction are fitted to the respective autocalibration point and the weights are calculated by solving the resulting linear system. In contrast to the GRAPPA weight calculation and reconstruction, neighboring k_x points are included.*

gorithm in its original form unsuitable for the reconstruction of images acquired with the Hilbert-Moore sequence.

4.1.4. MCMLI

The Multi-Column-Multi-LIne (MCMLI) [6] enhancement of the GRAPPA algorithm extends the reconstruction of missing points to two dimensions. The GRAPPA algorithm works for a fixed frequency encoding position k_x. That means that the missing point (k_x, k_y) is reconstructed using the acquired points $(k_x, k_y - m\Delta k_y)$. The MCMLI approach extends this reconstruction scheme to include neighboring column points $(k_x - n\Delta k_x)$ into the reconstruction:

$$S_u(k_x, k_y) = \sum_l \sum_n \sum_m w_{lu}(k_x - n\Delta k_x, k_y - m\Delta k_y) S_l(k_x - n\Delta k_x, k_y - m\Delta k_y) \quad (4.8)$$

For the calculation of the weights, a floating net based fit (FNF) has been introduced which looks for similar arrangements of acquired points in complete k-space. All similar arrangements are used for the calculation of the autocalibration weights which are later on used for the reconstruction. The limitation of this approach is its dependence on a fixed neighborhood pattern. This works well for trajectories like EPI but is unsuitable for the Hilbert-Moore sequence. Despite the self-similarity of the Hilbert-Moore trajectory,

4.2. Hilbert-Moore Reconstruction

The reconstruction algorithm used for the Hilbert-Moore sequence is an autocalibrating enhancement of the PARS algorithm inspired by the MCMLI algorithm. The self-similarity of the Hilbert-Moore space filling curve is exploited to combine the autocalibration of GRAPPA, the k-space locality of PARS, and the multi-neighbor model of the MCMLI algorithm. The Hilbert-Moore reconstruction algorithm uses neighborhood relations inside a quadratic window centered in the point to be reconstructed to calculate the autocalibration weights which are needed for the reconstruction.

For each missing point (k_x, k_y), the algorithm inspects its direct neighbors shown in figure 4.6. For each neighborhood relation between the missing point (k_x, k_y) and its adjacent point (k'_x, k'_y) (i.e. all eight combinations like (k_x, k_y) and $(k_x, k_y - \Delta k_y)$ etc.), all acquired pairs (s,r) of points with the same neighborhood relation within the nxn window centered in (k_x, k_y) are selected. An example is shown in figure 4.7 for the relation (k_x, k_y) to $(k_x, k_y - \Delta k_y)$

According to the GRAPPA formalism (equation (4.7)), the points are assembled into matrices S for the source and R for the reference points, respectively. Using the relation described in equation (4.7), the coil combination matrix is calculated. After the weights have been calculated for all possible neighborhood relations (e.g. up, up-right, down, down-right in figure 4.6), the one expressing the least error during the weight calculation $e = |R - SW|$ is selected for reconstructing the missing point.

Standard border handling conditions (*zerofilling,mirror border handling,periodic border handling*) have been implemented for points near the edges of the acquired k-space matrix.

The sliding window used to select the points for the reconstruction can be compared to a rectangular filter on the data. The hard borders introduced by the sliding window led to artifacts within the image. Weighting the window with a Hanning filter (figure 4.8) leads to smoother images with less artifacts.

4. Image Reconstruction

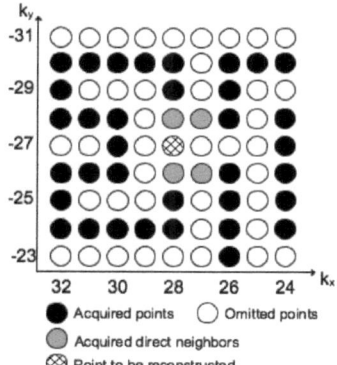

Figure 4.6.: *Direct neighborhood of a point to be reconstructed depicted in gray. Black dots represent the acquired trajectory. Window size 9×9*

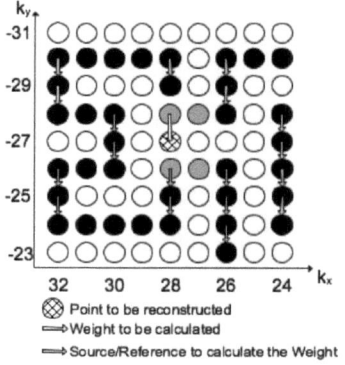

Figure 4.7.: *Source and reference (target) points in a 9x9 window used for the weights calculation for one possible neighbor relation.*

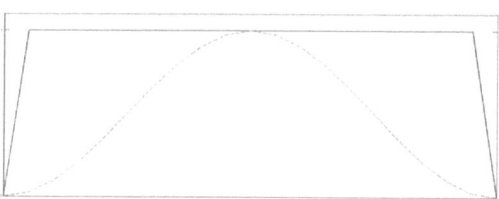

Figure 4.8.: *Hanning-Window (stippled line) and the rectangular window function (solid line)*

4. Image Reconstruction

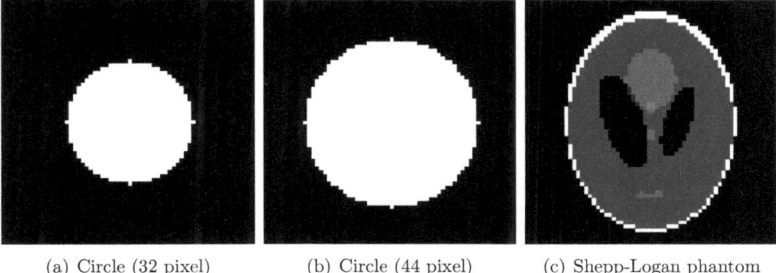

(a) Circle (32 pixel)   (b) Circle (44 pixel)   (c) Shepp-Logan phantom

Figure 4.9.: *Objects used for the simulation of the image reconstruction for the Hilbert-Moore sequence*

4.3. Results

The results for the image reconstruction algorithm are divided into two parts. In the first part, results from simulations are shown. This involves the reconstruction of three different objects for the estimation of the optimal window size and border condition. Five different simulation phantoms have been evaluated to estimate the optimal starting point of the Hilbert-Moore sequence.

In the second part, reconstruction of data acquired from the scanner is presented. This involves two different phantoms (a sphere and a quality phantom) and in-vivo brain images acquired from a volunteer. The different parameter combinations of the phantom measurements are given in table 4.1 on page 64.

4.3.1. Simulation

The reconstruction of the Hilbert-Moore sequence has been conducted for the three simulation objects shown in figure 4.9. To simulate the parallel acquisition with different coil sensitivities, four coil weightings with a randomized Gaussian profile have been used (figure 4.10).

Hanning filter

The influence of the Hanning filter window can be clearly seen in figure 4.11. The discontinuities introduced by the hard borders of the rectangular window disappear and

4. Image Reconstruction

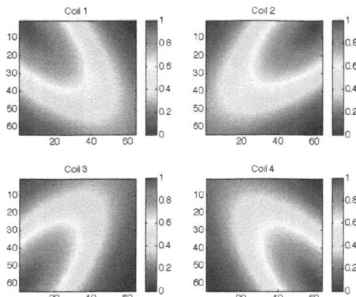

Figure 4.10.: *Simulation coil set based on a randomized two dimensional Gaussian curve centered at the edges*

a smoother image is reconstructed.

Variable Density Center Acquisition

Introducing gaps into the k-space matrix and reconstructing the image by calculation of the Fourier transformation without further processing leads to reconstruction artifacts, as shown in figure 4.12. By the application of the presented reconstruction algorithm, these artifacts can be reduced but are nevertheless clearly visible in the reconstructed image (figure 4.13).

The problem is the incorrectly reconstructed k-space center. In figure 4.14 the k-space center is shown as calculated by the reconstruction algorithm and originally sampled. To improve the image quality, additional dense sampling of the k-space center has been introduced (referred by variable density center). In figure 4.15 it is shown that image quality increases with increasing size of the variable density center region. The problem is that the additional dense sampling elongates the execution time of the sequence. The restriction to an 8x8 densely sampled k-space center region was the best compromise between image quality and sequence execution time.

4. Image Reconstruction

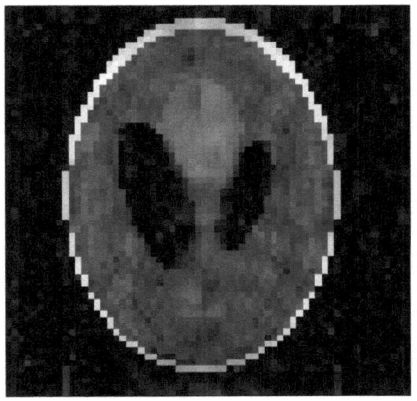
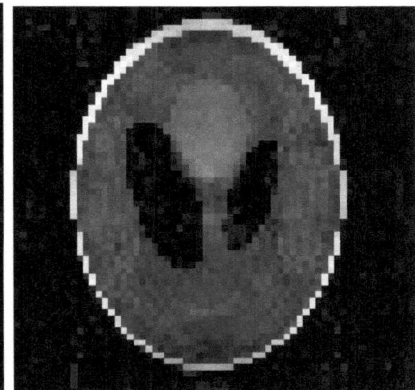

(a) Reconstruction with rectangular window

(b) Reconstruction with Hanning window

Figure 4.11.: *The hard borders of the rectangular window lead to discontinuities and artifacts in the reconstructed image (a). Weighting the window with the Hanning filter provides a smoother image (b) with less artifacts.*

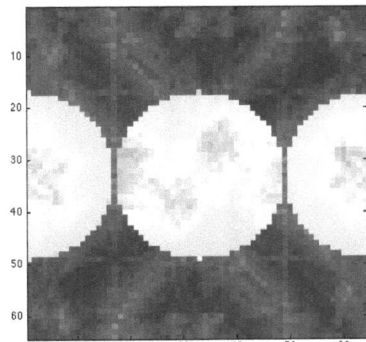
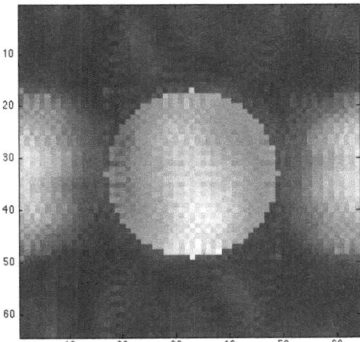

Figure 4.12.: *Reconstruction of a simulation phantom by taking the FFT of the acquired data*

Figure 4.13.: *Reconstruction of a simulation phantom with the application of the reconstruction algorithm*

4. Image Reconstruction

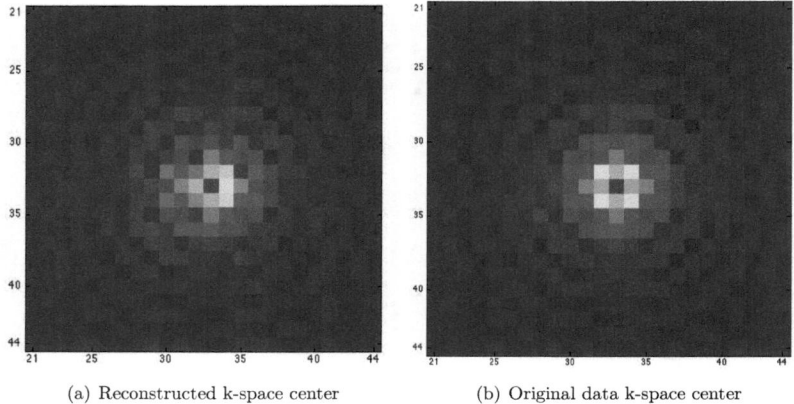

(a) Reconstructed k-space center (b) Original data k-space center

Figure 4.14.: *Comparison of reconstructed (a) and sampled (b) k-space center. Errors introduced by the reconstruction algorithm are clearly visible.*

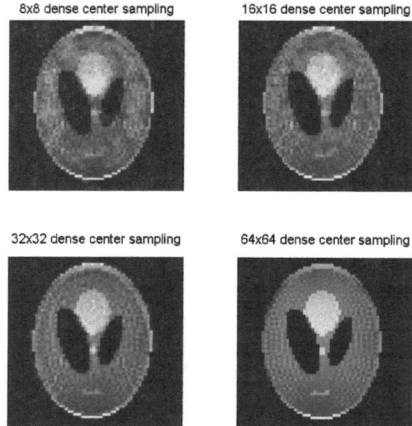

Figure 4.15.: *Different sizes of the densely sampled center. The image quality is proportional to the size of the variable density center. The 64x64 dense sampled center corresponds to the complete k-space matrix.*

4. Image Reconstruction

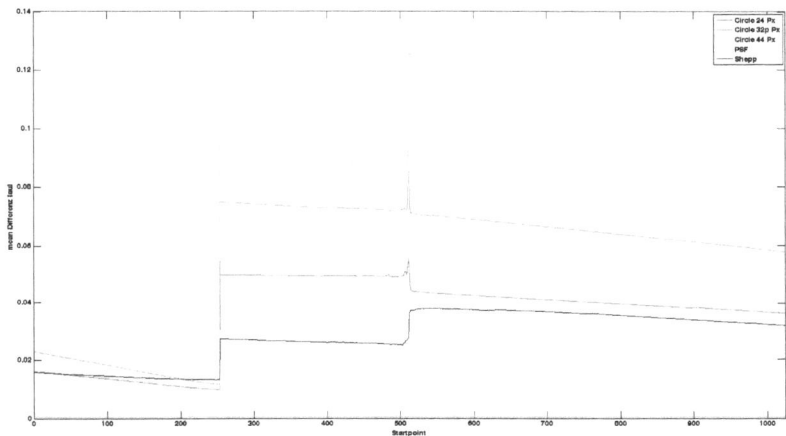

Figure 4.16.: *Estimation of the image quality of different starting points on the Hilbert-Moore trajectory for different simulation phantoms*

Optimal Starting Point

To estimate the optimal starting point, the Hilbert-Moore sequence is simulated with 5 different simulation phantoms and 1024 different starting points. A mono-exponential decay $e^{-\frac{t}{2094,2}}$ with t being the sampling step has been switched on during the starting point estimation. The value of 2094,2 has been found by a monoexponential fit of the signal decay acquired during a measurement of a sphere filled with tap water without any gradients switched on. As a quality criterion, the absolute difference between the starting point images and an image simulated without signal decay has been taken and the mean value over the complete difference image has been calculated. A plot of the mean difference versus the starting point is shown in figure 4.16. The images for the starting points with the minimum and the maximum difference as well as the images introducing the jump have been plotted in figure 4.17. The results for the best image quality are not really astonishing. Starting point 253 is the point where the variable density sampling scheme comes into play. Thus, the k-space center is sampled with most of the signal present. One step further, at starting point 254, the variable density sampling is executed at the end of the sequence, where most of the signal is gone. The

4. Image Reconstruction

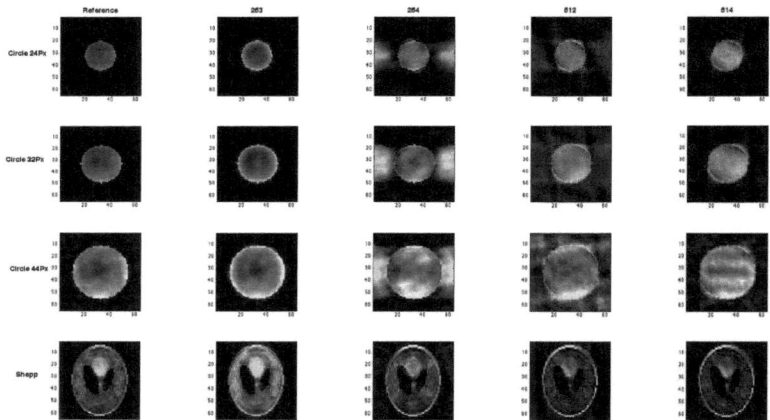

Figure 4.17.: *Reference, best (253) and worst (512/514) image estimated by the optimal starting point simulation. Also shown is the image that introduced the large jump in the graphs.*

worst image at point 512/513/514 can be explained very easily. Once again, the variable density k-space center is sampled very late in the sequence and in addition, the *time gap* (figure 3.17) between the left and the right side of k-space is very high, so that inconsistencies from this time gap have a very large influence. For the starting point at the opposite end (1024/1/2), this time gap is also present but here the variable density center has a much higher signal strength and thus compensates for the time gap.

Window Size and Border Handling Estimation

To estimate the optimal window size, the three simulation phantoms have been reconstructed using different window sizes and border handling conditions. The window sizes ranged from 7 (smallest size to find enough neighborhood relations) to 63 (nearly complete image). The resulting images have been normalized and subtracted from the original input data. The mean absolute value over the complete difference image has been used as a quality criterion. In figure 4.18 the mean difference curves are plotted for the three simulation phantoms. In figure 4.19 the reconstructed images are shown. The simulation results suggest that the influence of the border handling condition is negligible.

Figure 4.20 shows the complete reconstructed images for the window sizes for the Shepp Logan phantom. Visually there is no difference in the window sizes 19 to 29. In smaller window sizes the background of the Shepp Logan phantom becomes rippled. At window sizes above 29 the large circle in the upper part of the phantom gets distorted.

4.3.2. Scanner Phantom Data

Several datasets with different parameters have been acquired to evaluate the influence of e.g. FOV, gradient blip rise time, or the starting point. For most of these parameters, an EPI image with the same echo and repetition time has been acquired. For each EPI image, the GRAPPA acquisition has been turned on with the smallest number of reference lines possible (12) and a reduction factor of two, meaning that every second line has been left out. All datasets have been acquired with a 12-channel head coil on a Siemens TRIO 3T system at the Central Institute for Mental Health in Mannheim. The preface variable density sampling has proven to blur the image, so for the variable density acquired data, the inplace sampling method has been chosen. In addition to the

4. Image Reconstruction

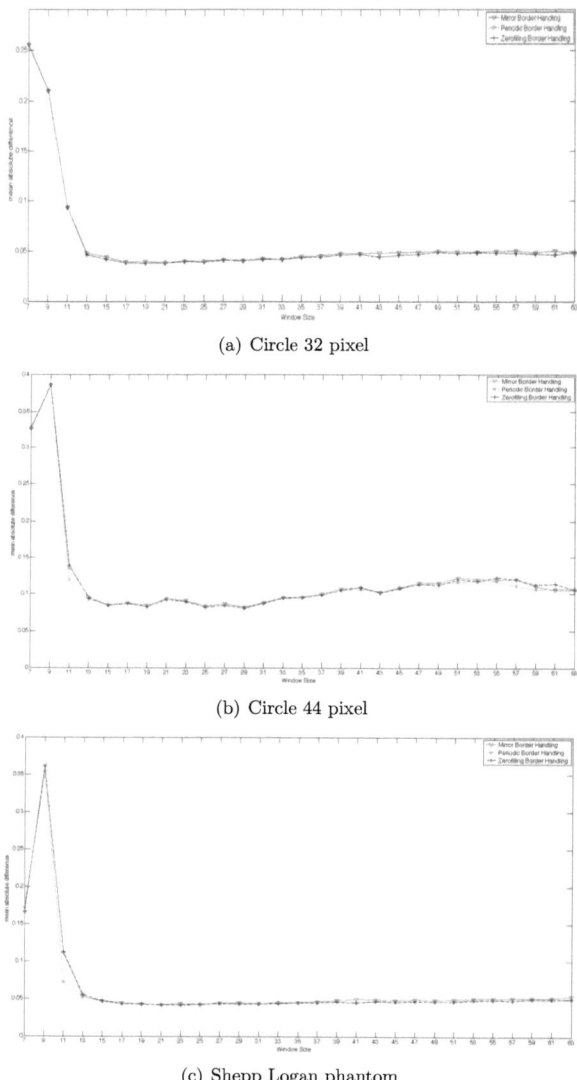

(a) Circle 32 pixel

(b) Circle 44 pixel

(c) Shepp Logan phantom

Figure 4.18.: *Mean absolute difference between original image and reconstructed image for different window sizes*

4. Image Reconstruction

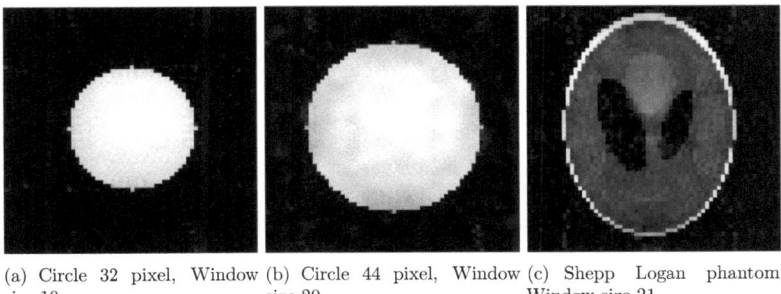

(a) Circle 32 pixel, Window size 19   (b) Circle 44 pixel, Window size 29   (c) Shepp Logan phantom, Window size 21

Figure 4.19.: *Reconstruction of the three simulation phantoms with the window size expressing the least mean absolute difference*

better image quality, the inplace sampling of the variable density data is consistent with the general understanding of echo time.

Risetime Modification and Field of View

In figure 4.21 the images for different fields of view and different rise times are shown. The reconstruction window size is 21 and the border condition is periodic border handling. The small cavity in the top part of the sphere is an air bubble inside the sphere. For all acquired fields of view, the outline of the sphere is clearly visible. Little artifacts distort the uniformity of the sphere. The elongated risetime reduces the overall signal strength (as expected) and introduces smearing artifacts for the threefold elongated rise time.

For all acquired fields of view, the Hilbert-Moore sequence provides acceptable image quality. The influence of the risetime modification is consistent for the different fields of view. Longer risetimes introduce artifacts due to the time-gap inherent in the Hilbert-Moore sequence sampling scheme. The uniformity of the sphere seems to improve with larger fields of view. This is due to the reduced detail quality seen in the smaller representations of the imaged object.

Starting point

The influence of the starting point (SP) is presented in figure 4.22. For the ultrashort echo time image with SP 253, smearing artifacts in the lower left corner or in the upper

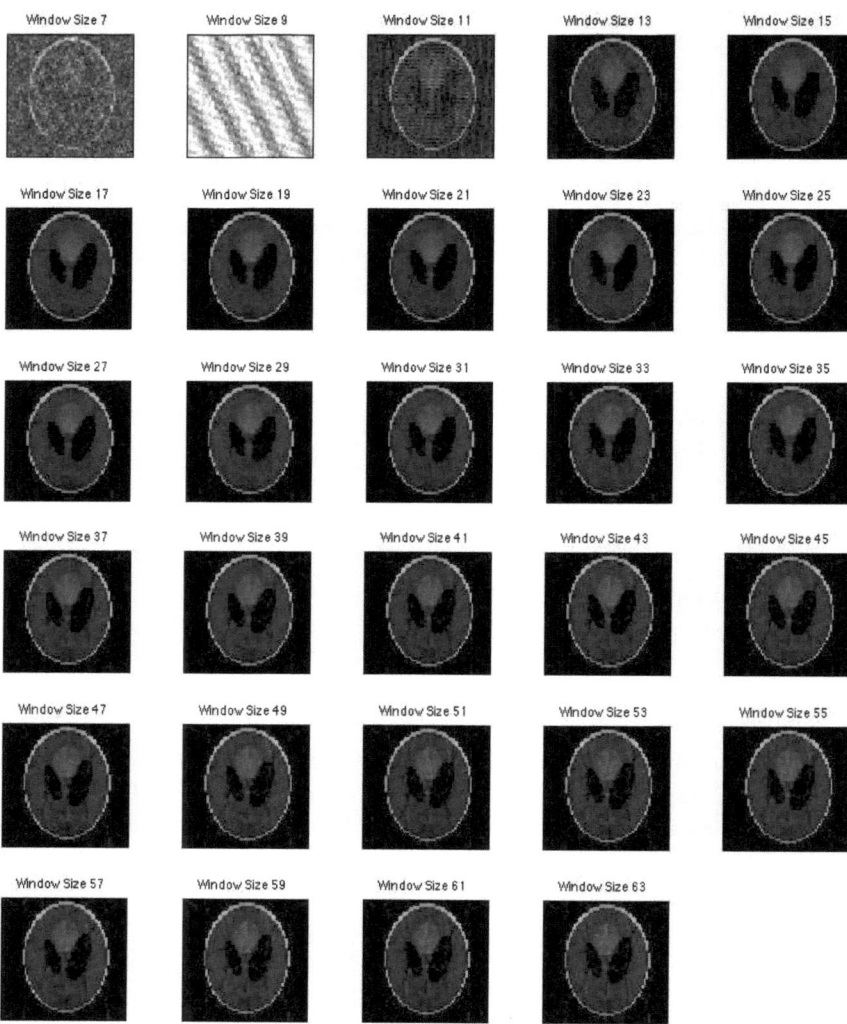

Figure 4.20.: *Reconstructions for the different window sizes for the Shepp-Logan Phantom*

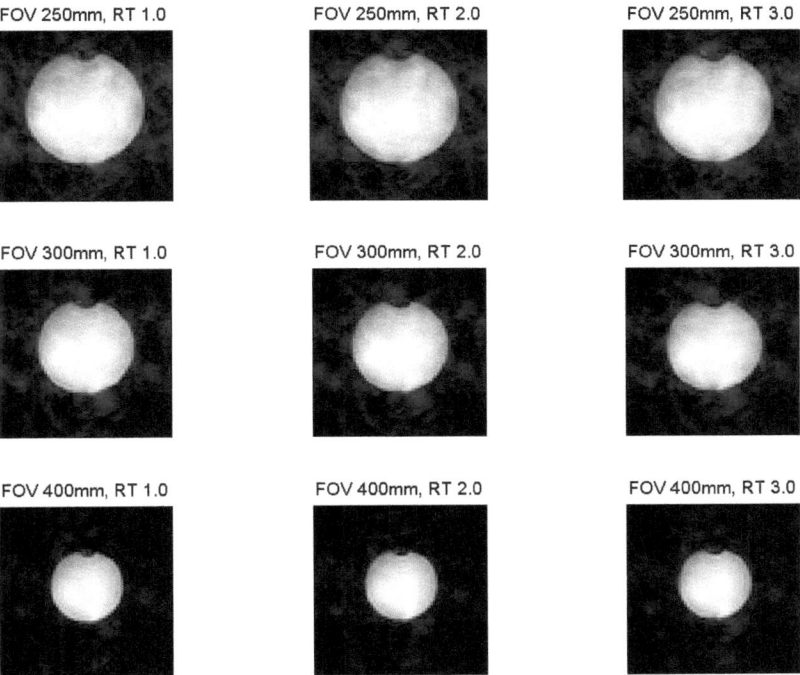

Figure 4.21.: *Overview of the acquired images for different fields of view and different rise time modificators*

4. Image Reconstruction

Table 4.1.: *Parameters of the acquired phantom data sets on the scanner. FOV is the field of view, risetime is the multiplication factor to elongate the minimal risetime, SP is the starting point, TE and TR the echo and the repetition time respectively. TE and TR are a direct consequence from the choice of the other parameters.*

Phantom	FOV [mm]	risetime	SP	TE [ms]	TR [ms]
Sphere/Quality	250	1.0	2	26	93
Sphere	250	2.0	2	33	114
Sphere	250	3.0	2	39	136
Sphere	300	1.0	2	26	93
Sphere	300	2.0	2	33	114
Sphere	300	3.0	2	39	136
Sphere	400	1.0	2	20	71
Sphere	400	2.0	2	26	92
Sphere	400	3.0	2	33	114
Sphere	250	1.0	253	6.2	93
Sphere	250	1.0	254/256	6	93
Sphere	250	1.0	512/513/514	67	93

part of the image are introduced. The large influence of the time gap is clearly visible for starting points 512 to 514. The uniformity is even more reduced (compared to the SP 2 images) and an artifact nearby the air bubble becomes clearly visible. For the longest echo time image with SP 256 (the center of the acquired k-space is SP 255), the influence of the signal decay and the time gap is very large. Distortions at the air bubble and a reduced uniformity can be clearly observed.

Reconstruction Window Size

To evaluate the influence of the window size and the border handling condition, the sphere and the quality phantom have been reconstructed with all possible combinations of border handling condition and window size. The signal-to-noise-ratio has been calculated and used as a quality criterion. In figure 4.23 the regions for the calculation of the signal-to-noise-ratio (SNR) for the sphere and the quality phantom are shown. The images have been normalized (respectively), and the two indicated 3×3 pixel regions have been selected. The mean value inside the regions has been calculated and the SNR has been estimated by the ratio of signal region to background region.

The resulting signal-to-noise-ratios for different window sizes and border handling

4. Image Reconstruction

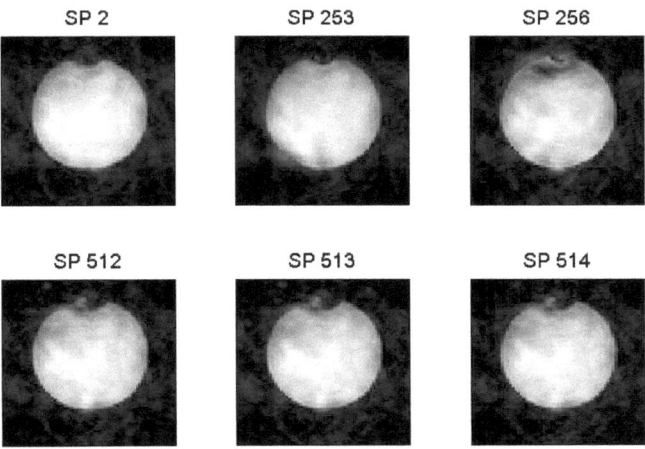

Figure 4.22.: *Overview of the acquired images for different starting points*

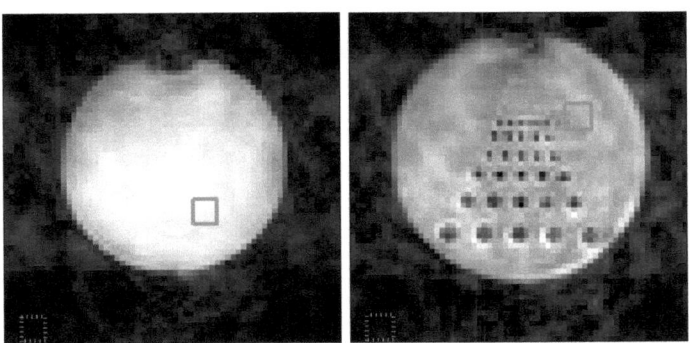

(a) Sphere Phantom SNR 38.26 WS 23 periodic border handling

(b) Quality Phantom SNR 12.91 WS 33 periodic border handling

Figure 4.23.: *SNR calculation for the sphere (a) and the quality phantom. The signal region is marked by the red box, the noise region by the stippled red box. Imaging parameters are a FOV of 250mm, a slice thickness of 2mm and SP 2 (TE=26ms, TR=93ms). The reconstruction window size (WS) and the border handling condition are indicated.*

4. Image Reconstruction

conditions are shown in figure 4.24. For small window sizes the SNR difference is minimal between the different border conditions. The influence of the border conditions is larger than suggested by the simulation but mainly the window size defines the image quality. Here the results are in good accordance with the simulation. Window sizes about 21 to 23 provide an acceptable signal-to-noise-ratio. For larger window sizes the SNR decreased for the sphere phantom but is still above a value of 20. For the quality phantom, the SNR is lower in general but also the variance in the SNR for larger window sizes is smoother.

Detail Resolution

The detail resolution of the quality phantom (figure 4.25 (a)) is quite acceptable for the image size of 64x64 pixels. The structure of the quality phantom can be distinguished up to the 6th line of points from a total of eleven lines in the phantom. This is quite comparable to the detail resolution provided by an EPI image (figure 4.25(b)) with the same TE, TR and FOV. For the EPI image, the standard GRAPPA reconstruction has been switched on and the minimum number of reference lines (12) in addition to a reduction factor of 2 has been selected.

In-Vivo Data

Figure 4.26 shows a series of brain images acquired with the Hilbert-Moore sequence. The detail resolution is limited by the image size of 64x64 pixels and the SNR of the Hilbert-Moore sequence. The main structures are nevertheless visible.

4.4. Discussion

The Hilbert-Moore sequence sampling pattern with the undersampling of k-space in frequency and phase-encoding direction renders standard parallel imaging reconstruction algorithms unusable. The newly developed Hilbert-Moore image reconstruction algorithm combines the autocalibration flexibility of GRAPPA with the k-space locality criterion of the PARS algorithm and the multidimensional reconstruction of the MCMLI algorithm.

The SNR and the image quality of the reconstructed images is mainly dependent on the window size. The best image quality is achieved with window sizes of about 21 to

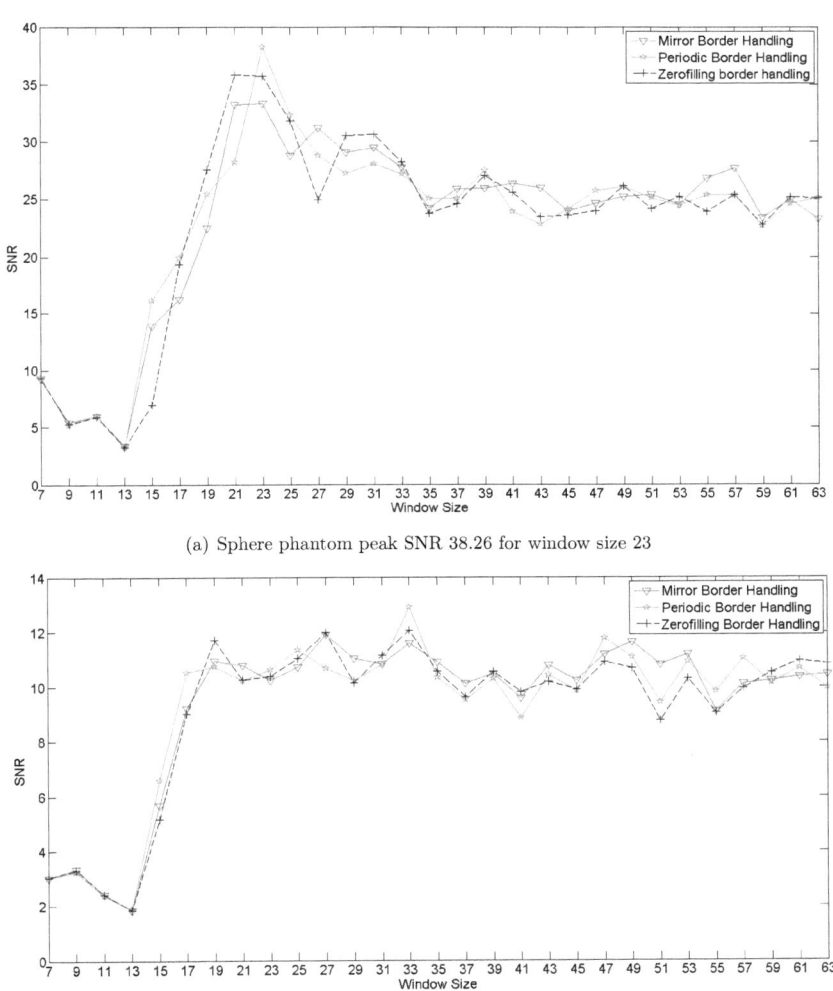

(a) Sphere phantom peak SNR 38.26 for window size 23

(b) Quality phantom peak SNR 12.91 for window size 33

Figure 4.24.: *signal-to-noise-ratios for different window sizes and border conditions evaluated for the Sphere and the Quality phantom. Imaging parameters: SP 2, TE 26ms, TR 93ms, FOV 250mm*

4. Image Reconstruction

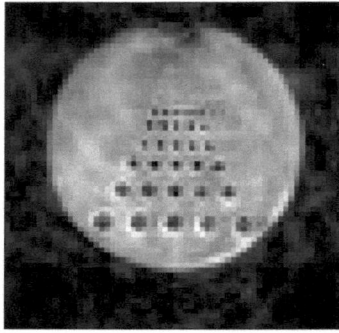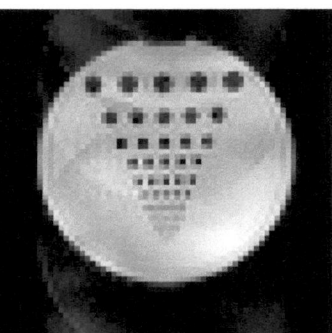

(a) Hilbert-Moore Sequence Quality Phantom (b) EPI Sequence Quality Phantom

Figure 4.25.: *Comparison between HM and EPI sequence quality phantom. Image parameters: FOV 250mm, TE 26ms, TR 93ms. The detail quality is comparable, but EPI provides better SNR*

25 pixels for the sphere or 33 for the quality phantom. For smaller window sizes the number of reference points is not sufficient to provide a good estimation of the weights used for the reconstruction. For larger window sizes, the influence of k-space points having a different signal strength than the point to be reconstructed becomes too large.

A prolongation of the rise time (and thus a longer TE and TR) does not necessarily distort the image quality. For the sphere phantom, it has been seen that the image quality for a doubled rise time is visually not differentiable. The choice of the starting point of the Hilbert-Moore sampling scheme proved to be quite important. The best image quality has been achieved with a starting point of 2, leading to a TE of 26 ms in combination with a rise time modifier of 1.0. The simulation of the optimal starting point proved to be unreliable. The image quality of the images with ultrashort echo times (suggested by the simulation) showed more artifacts than the images with a medium echo time. For the ultrashort echo times the differences in signal strength for neighboring points near the k-space center introduces artifacts. For long echo times, the data inconsistency introduced by the time gap inherent in the Hilbert-Moore sequence sampling scheme introduces even more artifacts.

The detail quality of the Hilbert-Moore images is quite comparable to the detail quality provided by a standard EPI sequence with the same imaging parameters. The SNR of

4. Image Reconstruction

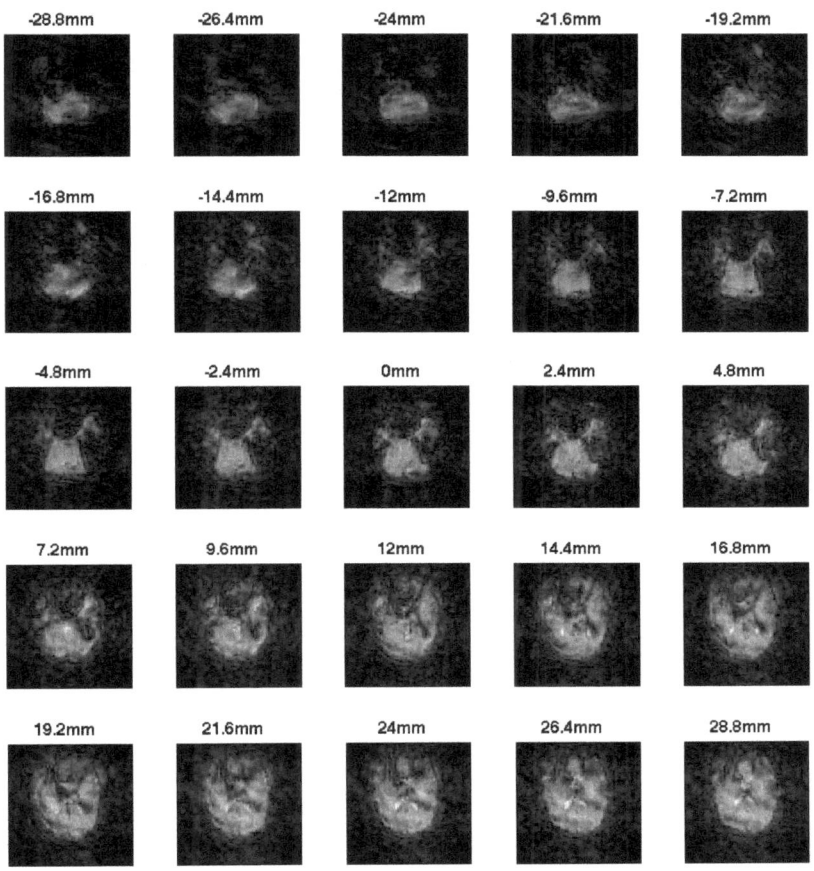

Figure 4.26.: *Overview of acquired slices of a volunteers brain. The slice positions are as indicated, 0mm is iso-center*

4. Image Reconstruction

the Hilber-Moore sequence images is lower than the SNR of EPI images with the same imaging parameters but still high enough to render the important structures visible.

Bibliography

[1] D. K. Sodickson and W. J. Manning. Simultaneous acquisition of spatial harmonics (SMASH): Fast imaging with radiofrequency coil arrays. *Magnetic Resonance in Medicine*, 38:591–603, 1997.

[2] K. P. Pruessmann, M. Weiger, M. B. Scheidegger, and P. Boesiger. SENSE: sensitivity encoding for fast MRI. *Magnetic Resonance in Medicine*, 42(5):952–962, 1999.

[3] M. A. Griswold, P. M. Jakob, R. M. Heidemann, M. Nittka, V. Jellus, J. Wang, B. Kiefer, and A. Haase. Generalized autocalibrating partially parallel acquisitions (GRAPPA). *Magnetic Resonance in Medicine*, 47:1202–1210, 2002.

[4] E. N. Yeh, C. A. McKenzie, D. Lim, M. A. Ohliger, A. K. Grant, J. D. Willig, N. Rofsky, and D. K. Sodickson. Parallel imaging with augmented radius in k-space (PARS). In *Proc. Intl. Soc. Mag. Reson. Med 10*, 2002.

[5] E. N. Yeh, C. A. McKenzie, M. A. Ohliger, and D. K. Sodickson. Parallel magnetic resonance imaging with adaptive radius in k-space (PARS): constrained image reconstruction using k-space locality in radiofrequency coil encoded data. *Magnetic Resonance in Medicine*, 53(6):1383–1392, 2005.

[6] Z. Wang, J. Wang, and J. A. Detre. Improved data reconstruction method for GRAPPA. *Magnetic Resonance in Medicine*, 54:738–742, 2005.

5. Sound

Over the last decades the trend to faster and even faster imaging sequences in conjunction with higher field strengths eclipsed the sound generated by the MR imager. Several publications on measuring the sound pressure level (SPL) have been presented (e.g. [1–5]) but no satisfactory solution to eliminate or reduce the acoustic noise has yet been found. The peak sound pressure level measured in a standard imaging experiment was in the range of 123 dB(A) to 138 dB(A) [6, 7], which is not only above the human pain threshold (120 dB(A)) but also above the officially recommended SPL in working environments.

The implications (section 5.1) and the generation (section 5.2) of acoustic noise in MR imagers are covered before some acoustic noise attenuation methods (section 5.3) are presented. In section 5.4 the sound measurement method used in this work is described. The last two sections cover the resulting acoustic noise for the Hilbert-Moore sequence (section 5.5) and the discussion of the results (section 5.6).

5.1. Implications

The acoustic noise generated by the MR imager is not only a health risk for patient and working staff but also a problem in functional MRI (fMRI), where brain activation mechanisms are investigated. In table 5.1 the mechanism of acoustic noise interference during fMRI is shown [8].

Especially in auditory fMRI (e.g. speech processing, tinnitus research), the acoustic noise generated by the MR scanner clearly influences the results and hinders communication between the subject and the researcher [9]. Several surveys have proven that the fMRI activity in the auditory cortex decreases for presented stimuli having similar frequencies as the MR scanner peak frequency [10–12].

In addition to the effects on auditory fMRI, several other implications of acoustic noise have been shown:

Table 5.1.: *Mechanisms of acoustic noise interference during fMRI [8]*

Mechanism	Characteristics
Direct confounding	
Intra-acquisition response	Activation by scanner noise within same volume acquisition
Inter-acquisition response	Activation by scanner noise of preceding volume acquisition
Indirect confounding	
Attention	Increased activation in attention-related cortical areas
Distraction	Decreased activation in cortical areas by (inter-modal) distraction
Habituation	Slowly developing adaptional loss of attention; might be advantageous in noisy environments
Motion artifacts	Not substantially related to scanner noise
Masking	Overlap of spectral components of scanner noise and auditory stimuli
Stapedial muscle reflex	Changes in cochlear perception of auditory stimuli (intensity and frequency)
Temporal hearing loss	Changes in cochlear perception of auditory stimuli (intensity and frequency)

- brain activation during a verbal memory task is increased with acoustic noise being present [13],

- cortical activity of the visual cortex decreased in combination with acoustic noise [14],

- for a delay of ~300ms between acoustic noise during fMRI acquisition and a single flash of light, the number of activated pixels in the visual cortex decreased significantly [15],

- cortical activation monitored by fMRI reflects the subjective perception rather than the physically present stimulus [16],

- the acoustic noise generated by the MR scanner reduces pain unpleasantness ratings compared to the same stimuli presented without acoustic noise [17].

All these findings show the urgent need for silent imaging sequences, especially in the context of fMRI research.

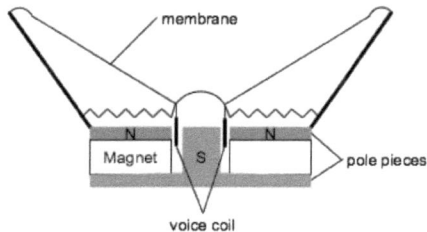

Figure 5.1.: *Schematic drawing of a conventional speaker*

5.2. Sound Generation

The sound generation in the MR imager follows the same mechanism as in a conventional speaker shown in figure 5.1. A current flowing through a wire inside a magnetic field induces vibrations. If the wire is connected to the surrounding material, the vibrations are transmitted to the material and finally to the air. Mansfield [18] explained the theory in more details, along with an examination of different materials for the supporting plates of the coil.

When supporting plates of plastic material are subjected to alternating transverse Lorentz forces while in a strong magnetic field normal to the plate surface, compressional waves within the solid produce a modulation of the plate surface that launches an acoustic wave in air along the magnetic field axis [18].

5.3. Noise Reduction Mechanisms

The efforts to reduce acoustic noise during MR imaging can be grouped into three independent classes. The first class is the physical modification of the scanner hardware. An overview of known approaches is given in section 5.3.1. This section also includes the efficacy of passive and active acoustic noise reduction at the subject side e.g. by the use of ear plugs. The second class is the optimization of imaging strategies, covering the design of an acoustic noise optimized fMRI experiment setup described in section 5.3.2. The last group is the optimization of existing pulse sequences. In section 5.3.3 the main optimization approaches for EPI and the FLASH sequence are presented.

5.3.1. Hardware Modifications

The major source of the acoustic noise during MR imaging are the gradient coils. It has been proposed to introduce additional windings that would quench sound propagation directly within the coil [19–22]. For these additional windings, a reduction of the SPL of about 30 dB has been reported.

Impeding the propagation of the acoustic wave from the coils to the surrounding material has been achieved by enclosing the coil in a vacuum chamber and mounting the gradient system to the floor instead of mounting it to the supporting material of the scanner [23, 24]. SPL reductions of up to 33 dB could be achieved with these approaches.

The most simple damping mechanism, the placement of sound isolating material inside the bore and near the shrouds [25], has been reported to achieve a noise reduction of about 18 dB.

A different source of acoustic noise, the acoustic noise generated by eddy currents in the supporting materials, has been tackled by mounting a passive metal shield on the outside of a vibration-isolated, vacuum-enclosed shielded gradient set [26]. A reduction of acoustic noise by about 26 dB has been reported for this approach.

In addition to reduction of the acoustic noise within and directly adjacent to the MR imager, a recommendation on the architectural design of a scanner room has been given [27] to reduce the annoyance of working staff in nearby offices.

The major drawback of all the hardware modifications presented before is the commercial unavailability. The MR scanner as an approved medical device cannot be modified at the site where it is placed due to the loss of its approval. On the other side, the hardware manufacturers are anxious to keep the production costs as low as possible. So the future, with the even higher field strengths will show if one or the other option to reduce acoustic noise by hardware modification will be available.

The most widely used acoustic noise reduction mechanism is the use of earplugs or earmuffs. This reduces the SPL arriving at the ears of the subject, but does not affect the generation of the acoustic noise. The attenuation achieved by using earplugs or earmuffs ranges from 5 to 38 dB [28] but depends on the frequency of the acoustic noise. Additional discomfort for the patient can be introduced and if the attenuators are not fitting perfectly, the effect is considerably reduced [29]. It has also been proposed to use a helmet or soft material surrounding the head to reduce the influence of bone conduction. This introduces not only additional discomfort but is furthermore unnecessary. It has been shown that bone conduction does not increase the perceived SPL during MR image acquisition [30].

Another option for noise reduction at the subject side is the use of Active Noise Cancellation (ANC). This equipment, well known to frequent flyers, records the noise in the environment and produces a sound wave that is opposite to the predominant noise wave and thus cancels it out. Unfortunately, none of the commercially existing products is known to be MR compatible, so this is still a field of ongoing research [31–33]. A degradation in image quality and safety concerns for the subject are the main problems with commercially available equipment. Another drawback is that this equipment does not work well for pulsed sound noise like generated by the EPI sequence.

Recently a string model to describe the vibrations in the MR coil [34] has been presented. The derived theoretical pulse sequence scheme [35, 36] that generates counter vibrations and therefore cancels the acoustic wave has not yet found its way into practical sequence design.

5.3.2. Imaging Strategies

The usual fMRI Block sequence design involves high repetition numbers and therefore a practically *continuous* scanning during the experiment. This may have the advantage that the subject habituates to the sound noise but on the other side, the auditory cortex during an acquisition is still influenced by the acoustic noise generated from the previous acquisition. To overcome the limitations of continuous sampling, a sparse sampling scheme has been proposed for auditory fMRI that acquires a single volume (instead of multiple volumes) at the end of the presented stimulus and at the end of the baseline condition [37, 38]. The newly proposed sparse sampling scheme resulted in higher activation signal from the regions of interest. A reduction of crossmodal effects (e.g. influence of the acoustic noise during visual stimulation experiments) and a higher attention level to the presented stimuli but no reduction of the sound pressure level of the acoustic noise can be achieved with this approach.

Acoustic noise reduction by parallel imaging is also possible. By reducing the amount of data acquired during a single scan and reconstructing the missing information afterwards by using reconstruction techniques like SMASH or SENSE, the acquisition time can be reduced. If the acquisition time is kept constant, the use of parallel imaging techniques allows to reduce the gradients slewrate and amplitude [39]. A reduction of the SPL of about 16 dB has been reported for this approach.

5.3.3. Acoustic Noise Optimizations for FLASH and EPI

The main optimization method for FLASH and EPI is the adjustment of the gradient waveform. It has been shown that *soft* (e.g. sinusoidal) waveforms have an advantage over the usually implemented trapezoidal waveforms in terms of acoustic noise [40–42]. The difficulty in using these sinusoidal waveforms lies in the resulting non-cartesian sampling pattern in addition with a non uniform distribution of the sampling points in k-space. This requires a large amount of post-processing algorithms like Gridding [43] and therefore a very accurate determination of the actual trajectory. In addition, the risk for peripheral nerve stimulation to occur during image acquisition is higher with sinusoidal waveforms [44].

Other optimization methods include the avoidance of mechanical resonance frequencies of the gradient coils [45] and the implementation of a quasi-continuous gradient switching pattern [46] to exploit the fact that the human auditory cortex is especially sensitive to pulsed sounds. Reduced BOLD activity during the rest-state and increased BOLD amplitude with stimuli present has been reported for the quasi-continuous gradient switching approach.

In a recent work [47] a reduction of the SPL of about 20 dB has been achieved by the combination of several proposed approaches for an EPI sequence:

- Avoiding mechanical resonance peaks [45],
- Using sinusoidal readout gradients [40, 41],
- Exploiting parallel imaging [39].

5.4. Sound Measurement

The first acoustic noise measurements have been conducted in cooperation with the Berufsgenossenschaft Nahrungsmittel und Gaststätten. Their equipment proved to be unusable in the strong magnetic environment. Even with a dummy head instead of a microphone, values of about 80 dB(A) for a standard imaging sequence have been measured. In the following, the measurement setup used in this work (similar to the one used in [3]) is described.

5.4.1. Equipment

To keep the influence of the main magnetic field as low as possible, a small electret condenser microphone (Ringford CZ034 Series) has been used. The microphone was connected via a 10m shielded cable to a pre-amplifier from LC Electronic powered by a 9V block battery. Using the external sound card *Instant Music* from ADS Tech[1], the preamplifier was connected via USB port to an Apple iBook G4 (running on battery during measurements) and the freeware Audacity[2] was used to sample the input recorded by the microphone using a sampling frequency of 44.1 kHz and a sample format of 32bit float. To resolve frequencies higher than 5000Hz, the option *High Quality Sinc Interpolation* with *Shaped* dithering has been chosen. The recorded data has been saved as a WAV (Microsoft 32 bit float PCM) file. The resulting file has been loaded into MATLAB (The Mathworks Inc.) for further processing.

5.4.2. Microphone Calibration

The calibration of the recording system has been done in an anechoic chamber used for hearing tests at the University Hospital of Mannheim. Several tunes of defined frequency and Sound Pressure Level (SPL) (table 5.2) have been recorded.The head of the microphone was placed within 20cm distance to a free field speaker with a 110° degree angle of reflected beam. The cable was laid in curves so that no crossings occurred. The sound started playing before the recording started and stopped after the recording has been finished. From the recorded 10 seconds a fragment of length 1 second has been cut out in the middle of the recording for further analysis. Several measurements (marked with an O in table 5.2) are out of the dynamic range of the measuring equipment. A comparison with nearby measurements of the frequencies in question showed no difference in the amplitude values. For the 1000 Hz tune more calibration tunes have been measured because 1000Hz is the reference frequency for several calculations in audio processing ([48]).

The one second fragments are loaded into MATLAB and a Fast Fourier Transformation (FFT) is applied to obtain the frequency spectrum. The sampling frequency of 44100 Hz leads to a frequency range of 0 Hz to 22050 Hz. The software used to control the hearing test equipment in the University Hospital in Mannheim was limited to the

---
[1] http://www.adstech.com
[2] http://audacity.sourceforge.net

Table 5.2.: *Sound Pressure Levels in dB(A) and frequencies [Hz] measurement for the Microphone calibration. Measurements marked with O are out of the dynamic range of the measuring equipment. Measurements without any mark were not possible with the tune playing equipment. The octave band filter middle frequencies (according to DIN 45651) are marked in* **bold** *font.*

Hz	50	55	60	65	70	75	80	85	90	95	100	105	110
125	X		X		X	O							
250	X		X		X	X	X		O		O		
500	X		X		X	X	X		X		O		
750	X		X		X	X	X		X		O	O	
1000	X	X	X	X	X	X	X	X	X	O	O	O	O
1500	X		X		X	X	X		X		X	X	X
2000	X		X		X	X	X		X		X	O	O
3000	X		X		X	X	X		X		X	X	X
4000	X		X		X	X	X		X		X	X	X
6000	X		X		X	X	X		X		O	O	O
8000	X		X		X	X	X		X		O		
10000	X		X		X	X	X		X				

frequencies measured (table 5.2). Most of these frequencies are the standard middle frequencies of the octave band filters defined in DIN 45651. An octave band filter is a filter that has relative bandwidth and its cut-off frequencies (f_l for lower and f_u for upper) can be calculated from the middle frequency f_m by using equation (5.1). The representative amplitude for an octave band is found by calculating the root-mean-square of the amplitude for the different frequencies covered by the bandwidth.

$$\begin{aligned} f_l &= \tfrac{1}{\sqrt{2}} \cdot f_m \\ f_u &= \sqrt{2} \cdot f_m. \end{aligned} \quad (5.1)$$

For each calibration tune, the octave band for the corresponding middle frequency is calculated. In a second step, the A-correction for the SPL values is removed and a spline interpolation is done over the SPL range covered by the calibration tunes. The results are shown in table B.1 which is further used as a lookup table between amplitude and frequency to determine the SPL for the following measurements.

5.4.3. Measurement Setup

The sound of the MR imager has been measured in different sessions. The microphone and the cable have been fed through a cable channel from the control room to the magnet room. The microphone has been fixed onto a standard sphere phantom inside the twelve-channel head coil available at the Siemens TIM Trio System. The tip of the microphone was positioned at the iso-center of the magnet. A standard EPI sequence with a flip angle of $10°$ and the Hilbert-Moore sequence with a flip angle of $5°$ have been measured for a variety of parameters. The influences of the starting point, the field of view (FOV), the repetition time (TR), the slewrate, and the gradient axis have been evaluated. For a certain number of parameters, a standard EPI sequence with the same main imaging parameters (FOV, TE, TR) has been measured. At the start of each measurement session, a reference measurement has been performed to check for low battery power for the amplifier, different hardware settings, and other equipment influences.

5.4.4. Data Evaluation

Before the acquired data is loaded into MATLAB (The Mathworks Inc.) for further processing, a fragment of length one second is cut out in the middle of the recording and saved as a separate WAV file. If the repetition time is long enough to distinguish single sequence executions, the mask is placed so that a single measurement lies completely inside the one second fragment. The stored one second fragment is loaded into MATLAB afterwards, and the octave band values are calculated as described in section 5.4.2. The amplitude values are then looked up in table B.1 and the resulting sound pressure level is rounded to the next higher value. The overall sound pressure level of the sequence is determined by the root mean squared (RMS) value of the SPL values of the individual octave bands.

5.5. Results

5.5.1. Calibration

Figure 5.2 shows the measured calibration values, fitted with a B-spline to fill the complete dynamic range of the calibration measurement. In the appendix, in table B.1 the

5. Sound

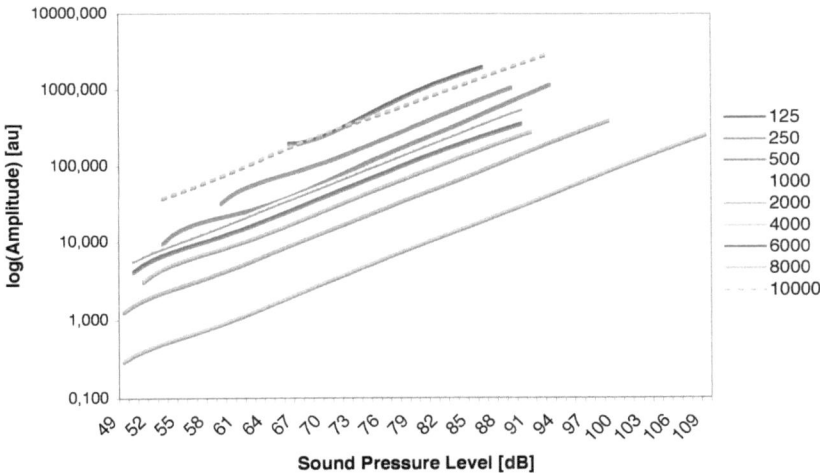

Figure 5.2.: *Plot of the (logarithmic) amplitude versus the Sound Pressure level in dB for the different frequencies (given in Hz).*

numerical values are shown. In the following these values are used as a lookup table to estimate the SPL in dB from the measured amplitudes.

5.5.2. Imaging Sequences

In table 5.3 some of the measured sound pressure levels for the main imaging parameters used in fMRI are shown. The overall sound energy transmitted by the Hilbert-Moore

Table 5.3.: *Sound pressure levels measured for the main sequence parameters. Shown are the octave band filter results, and the overall (root mean squared, RMS) loudness with A-level correction applied, for a continuous measurement of multiple slices. Differences from the mean value (if any) are as indicated.*

Seq Parameters (FOV TR TE)	RMS [dB(A)]	500Hz [dB]	1kHz [dB]	2kHz [dB]	3kHz [dB]	4kHz [dB]	6kHz [dB]	8kHz [dB]	10kHz [dB]
EPI 194 92 26	77	61	76	84+1	95	89	65	66	74
HM 194 92 26	83	58	68-1	87	100	99	78	80	86
EPI 250 92 26	75	58	74	84	94+1	89	64-1	63	71
HM 250 93 26	80	56	65±1	85	98	97	75	77	83
EPI 300 93 26	74	58	72	82	93	89	63	62	67+1
HM 300 93 26	79	55	64	84	96	95	74	76	82

sequence is higher than the overall sound energy transmitted by an EPI sequence with comparable parameters TE and TR. This emerges from the high sound energy levels transmitted in the octave bands for frequencies above 2 kHz. In the octave bands below 2 kHz, the Hilbert-Moore sequence transmits less sound energy to its environment than a comparable EPI sequence. This can be seen more clearly in figure 5.3, where the acoustic noise transmitted by the Hilbert-Moore sequence and the EPI sequence is shown as a frequency plot. Moreover, figure 5.3 shows that the Hilbert-Moore sequence covers a broader range of frequencies in contrast to the EPI sequence which has distinct dominant peak frequencies. This leads to a different acoustic noise characteristic. The EPI sequence acoustic noise for the executed continuous multi slice measurement is perceived as multiple pulsed tones, one for each measured slice. The Hilbert-Moore frequency acoustic noise is perceived as a buzzing sound, resembling to white noise, for each measured slice.

In the following, the influence of different imaging parameters on the acoustic noise generated by the Hilbert-Moore sequence is presented.

5. Sound

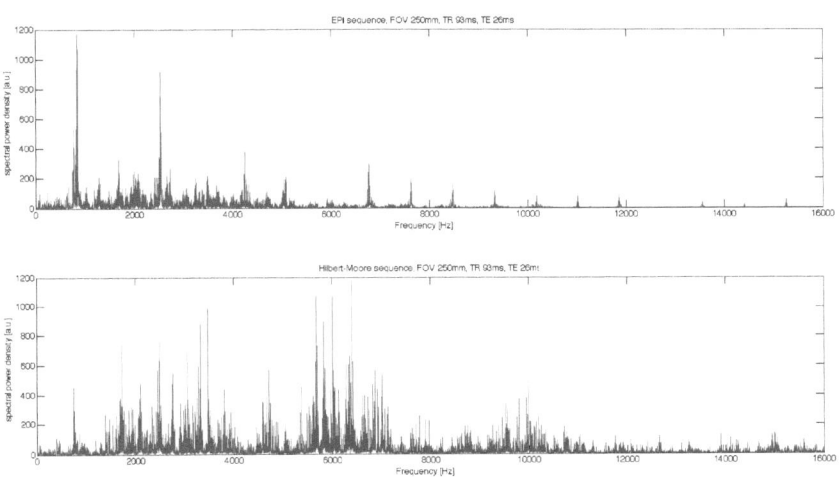

Figure 5.3.: *Frequency plot of the acoustic noise for the EPI (upper) and the HM (lower) sequence.*

FOV

Table 5.4.: *Hilbert-Moore sequence SPL for different FOV. Differences from the mean value are indicated.*

FOV [mm]	TR [ms]	TE [ms]	RMS [dB(A)]	500Hz [dB]	1kHz [dB]	2kHz [dB]	3kHz [dB]	4kHz [dB]	6kHz [dB]	8kHz [dB]	10kHz [dB]
194	92	26	**83**	58	68-1	87	100	99	78	80	86
250	93	26	**80**	56	65±1	85	98	97	75	77	83
300	93	26	**79**	55	64	84	96	95	74	76	82
350	71	20	**80**	54	65	83	99	99	72	74	86
400	71	22	**79**	54	64	82	97+1	97	71	73	84

Table 5.4 shows the acquired sound pressure levels for different fields of view. It can be seen that the overall sound pressure level does not depend directly on the FOV. A clear reduction of the overall sound pressure level can only be observed for the enlargement of the FOV from 194 to 250 mm. A reduction of the SPL over the complete frequency range can be observed for this step.

5. Sound

For the step from a FOV of 300 to 350mm which goes along with a change in the TR and TE, a shift of the sound energy can be seen in table 5.4. The reduction in TR and TE indicates a higher gradient switching speed due to lower gradient peak amplitudes, which leads to shorter rise times for the triangular blip-edges. The higher gradient switching can be observed in the shift of the sound energy to higher frequency regions. The sound pressure level for the octave band of 500 Hz is reduced considerably and the sound energy of the 3000 Hz and 4000 Hz octave bands is increased.

TR variation

Table 5.5.: *Hilbert-Moore sequence SPL for different TR, a TE of 26ms and a FOV of 250mm. Differences from the mean value are indicated.*

TR [ms]	RMS [dB(A)]	500Hz [dB]	1kHz [dB]	2kHz [dB]	3kHz [dB]	4kHz [dB]	6kHz [dB]	8kHz [dB]	10kHz [dB]
93	80	56	65±1	85	98	97	75	77	83
150	78	54	64	83	95+1	95	73	75	81
300	79	<53	61+1	80±1	92+1	92±1	70+1	72+1	77+2
1000	74	<53	56	75	87-1	87	65	67	72
3000	73	<53	56	74	88	87	65	67	70

For rising TR, the sound pressure level decreases in each frequency band. For a TR of 1000ms and a TR of 3000ms, practically no difference in the sound pressure levels can be observed for the HM measurements. During data analysis a fragment of length one second is cut out of the complete acoustic noise recording. For these two TR, a single slice measurement fits into the data fragment. The overall behavior of the sound pressure level stays consistent for the different TR. The sound energy is rising until it reaches its peak in the frequency band of 3000 Hz and 4000 Hz, drops for the following two frequency bands and rises again in the 10 kHz frequency band. In figure 5.4 the overlaid frequency plots for the Hilbert-Moore sequence are shown. It can be seen that the frequency distribution stays the same for the different repetition times; only the amplitude changes. This suggests that for shorter TR the acoustic noise generated by the previously measured slices has a large influence on the sound pressure level of the actual slice due to transient oscillations.

5. Sound

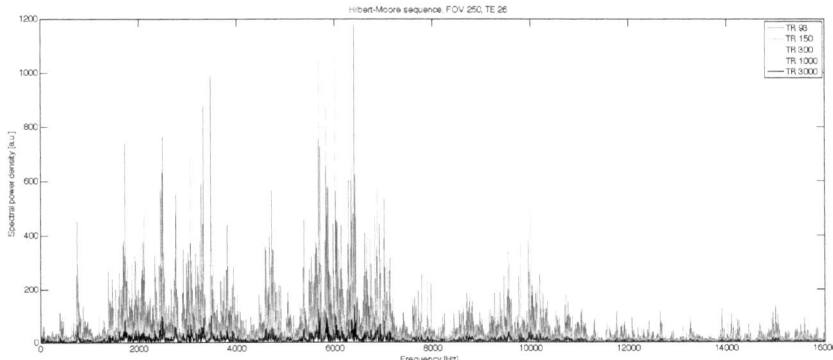

Figure 5.4.: *Overlay frequency plot for the Hilbert-Moore sequence with different repetition times. The frequency distribution does not change, only the amplitude decreases for longer TR.*

Starting Point Variation

The influence of the preparation gradients on the acoustic noise has been evaluated by changing the starting point of the Hilbert-Moore sequence. In table 5.6 the sound pressure levels for the different starting points are listed. The preparation gradient has practically no impact on the acoustic noise of the Hilbert-Moore sequence. Even if both preparation gradients are played out to the maximum (lower left corner/upper right corner of covered k-space), the acoustic noise generated by the Hilbert-Moore sequence does not change considerably.

Slewrate Modification

Different rise times for the individual gradient blips change the slewrate, the repetition time, and the echo time. In table 5.7 the SPLs for different rise times in addition to the resulting TR and TE are shown. A decrease of the sound pressure levels especially in the high octave band frequencies can be observed. The frequency-plots in figure 5.5 for the different echo times achieved by the rise time factors confirm the observation. A clear shift of the energy present in the frequencies above 6000 Hz to lower frequencies can be observed. In reverse, this leads to the assumption that (if not hindered by gradient

Table 5.6.: *SPL for different start points of the Hilbert-Moore frequency to evaluate the influence of the preparation gradients. For the 500 Hz octave band filter all measurements result in values smaller than 53 dB for most measurements and is thus omitted here. The TR has been set to 1000ms to exclude the effect of transient oscillations.*

SP	(k_x, k_y)	RMS [dB(A)]	1kHz [dB]	2kHz [dB]	3kHz [dB]	4kHz [dB]	6kHz [dB]	8kHz [dB]	10kHz [dB]
2	(-2,-28)	**73**	56	74	87	87	65	67	72
32	(-8,-22)	**73**	55	74	87	86	65	67	72
48	(-14,-24)	**73**	55	74	87	86	65	67	72
85	(-30,-30)	**73**	56	75	87	87	65	67	72
127	(-16,-16)	**73**	55	74	87	87	65	67	72
149	(-30,-14)	**73**	55	74	87	86	65	67	72
170	(-30,0)	**73**	55	74	87	86	65	67	72
250	(-6,0)	**73**	55	73	86	86	65	67	72
341	(-30,2)	**73**	55	74	87	86	65	67	72
597	(32,32)	**73**	56	75	87	87	65	67	72

Table 5.7.: *The effect of different rise times on the SPL of the Hilbert-Moore sequence. For all measurements, a FOV of 250mm and a TR of 1000ms has been set. The starting point has been point 2. The SPL for the 500Hz octave band filter was below 53 dB for most measurements and is thus omitted here. RT is the Risetime multiplication factor. Differences from the mean value are marked.*

RT	TE [ms]	RMS [dB(A)]	1kHz [dB]	2kHz [dB]	3kHz [dB]	4kHz [dB]	6kHz [dB]	8kHz [dB]	10kHz [dB]
1.0	26	**73**	56	75	87	87-1	65	67	72
1.4	26	**73**	54	74	87	87	65	67	72
1.5	33	**72**	52	75	85	86	63	64	74
2.2	33	**72**	52	75	85	86	63	64	74
2.3	39	**71**	51	73	84	86	64	65	70
3.2	39	**71**	51	73	85	86	64	65	70
3.3	46	**71**	53	71	86	87	63	63	67
4.4	46	**71**	53	71	86	87	62	63	67

5. Sound

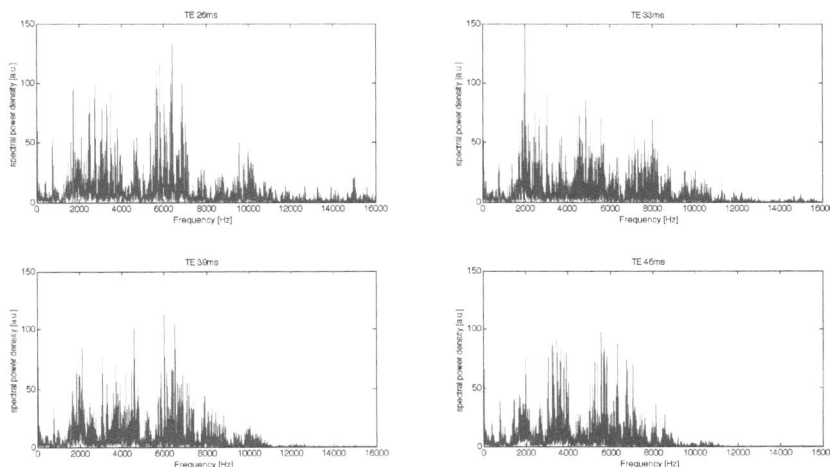

Figure 5.5.: *Variations in SPL for different rise times of the gradient blips. The correspondence between TE and the rise time modification can be found in table 5.7. Imaging parameters: FOV 250mm, TR 1000ms, Startpoint 2*

hardware limitations) faster switching of the gradient blips would shift the main sound energy even higher up in the frequency spectrum and possibly above the human hearing threshold.

Gradient Axes

In table 5.8 the acoustic noise resulting from a single gradient axis (by switching off gradients on other axes) is shown. Interestingly the sound pressure level depends on the gradient axes. For every measured TR, a difference between the two gradient axis can be seen. Especially for the octave bands of 2kHz to 6kHz, the y-gradient axis emits higher sound pressure levels than the x-gradient axis. The Hilbert-Moore sequence spreads gradient activity equally on both gradient axis so the load of the gradient axis should be equal and the same sound pressure level has been expected for both gradient axes.

Table 5.8.: *SPL for single gradient axes compared to the overall SPL of the complete measurement sequence. All measurements have been executed with a FOV of 250mm.*

TR [ms]	TE [ms]	Axis	**RMS [dB(A)]**	500Hz [dB]	1kHz [dB]	2kHz [dB]	3kHz [dB]	4kHz [dB]	6kHz [dB]	8kHz [dB]	10kHz [dB]
92	26	All	**80**	55	65	86	97+1	96	74	76	84
92	26	RO	**77**	58	65	81	92	92	72	74	80
92	26	PE	**78**	59	65	85	97	95	70	72	80
1000	26	All	**73**	<53	54	75	87	86	64	66	72
1000	26	RO	**70**	<53	54	71	82	81	62	64	69
1000	26	PE	**70**	<53	53	74	86	84	60	62	69
3000	26	All	**73**	<53	56	74	88	87	65	67	70
3000	26	RO	**69**	<53	54	69	82	82	61	63	66
3000	26	PE	**72**	<53	56	74	88	87	64	65	66

5.6. Discussion

The acoustic noise generated by the Hilbert-Moore sequence is completely different to the acoustic noise generated by the EPI sequence. The high number of gradient switchings and the feigned stochastic switching pattern leads to a broader frequency distribution of the sound energy. The resulting acoustic noise is smoother than the EPI sequence with its sharp pulsed sounds. For the human hearing system being very sensitive to pulsed sounds, the Hilbert-Moore sequence provides a more comfortable acoustic noise characteristic.

Regarding the overall sound pressure level of the two sequences in direct comparison, EPI seems to have an advantage of a few decibel. This advantage backs out when the octave band frequencies are analyzed. EPI provides higher sound pressure levels in the frequency range below 3000 Hz, whereas the Hilbert-Moore sequence provides higher sound pressure levels for frequencies above 4000 Hz. The efficacy of acoustic noise attenuators like earplugs increases for higher frequencies and therefore the acoustic noise generated by the Hilbert-Moore sequence can be better damped. In table 5.9 attenuation values from the literature [28] are applied to the results of the measurements. The original difference between the sound pressure level of EPI and the Hilbert-Moore sequence is halved, and the overall sound pressure level is reduced to under 60 dB for both sequences.

The gradient hardware, optimized for EPI (or other) sequences with the main gradient

Table 5.9.: *Comparison of the measured and the (theoretically) damped sound pressure levels*

Seq Parameters (FOV TR TE)	RMS [dB(A)]	**damped [dB(A)]**	500Hz [dB(A)]	1kHz [dB(A)]	2kHz [dB(A)]	4kHz [dB(A)]	8kHz [dB(A)]
Damping			15	16	10	26	38
EPI 194 92 26	77	**56**	43	60	75	64	27
HM 194 92 26	83	**59**	40	52	78	74	41
EPI 250 92 26	75	**55**	40	58	75	64	24
HM 250 93 26	80	**57**	38	49	76	72	38
EPI 300 93 26	74	**54**	40	56	73	64	23
HM 300 93 26	79	**56**	37	48	75	70	37

load on the x-gradient axis, makes it difficult for the Hilbert-Moore sequence to show its complete potential. The analysis of the sound pressure level generated by the individual gradient axis suggests that the damping of the x-gradient axis is more effective than the damping of the y-gradient axis. With better damping of the y-gradient axis and faster slew rates or gradient switching times the Hilbert-Moore sequence should show a clear advantage over the EPI sequence in matters of acoustic noise. Even with todays hardware, the Hilbert-Moore sequence acoustic noise is more pleasant for the human hearing system than the acoustic noise generated by an EPI sequence.

Bibliography

[1] Z. H. Cho, S. H. Park, J. H. Kim, S. C. Chung, S. T. Chung, J. Y. Chung, C. W. Moon, J. H. Yi, C. H. Sin, and E. K. Wong. Analysis of acoustic noise in MRI. *Magnetic Resonance Imaging*, 15:815–822, 1997.

[2] S. A. Counter, A. Olofsson, H. F. Grahn, and E. Borg. MRI acoustic noise: sound pressure and frequency analysis. *Journal of Magnetic Resonance Imaging*, 7:606–611, 1997.

[3] M. Knörgen, R. P. Spielmann, E. J. Haberland, and G. Melkus. Schalldruckpegelmessungen an einer MRT-anlage. *Zeitschrift für Medizinische Physik*, 14:251–259, 2004.

[4] G. Morton and C. Gildersleve. Noise in the MRI scanner. *Anaesthesia*, 55:1213, 2000.

[5] R. A. Hedeen and W. A. Edelstein. Characterization and prediction of gradient acoustic noise in MR imagers. *Magnetic Resonance in Medicine*, 37:7–10, 1997.

[6] J. R. Foster, D. A. Hall, A. Q. Summerfield, A. R. Palmer, and R. W. Bowtell. Sound-level measurements and calculations of safe noise dosage during EPI at 3T. *Journal of Magnetic Resonance Imaging*, 12(1):157–163, 2000 Jul.

[7] M. E. Ravicz, J. R. Melcher, and N. Y-S. Kiang. Acoustic noise during functional magnetic resonance imaging. *Journal of the Acoustical Society of America*, 108(4):1683–1696, 2000.

[8] A. Moelker and P. M. T. Pattynama. Acoustic noise concerns in functional magnetic resonance imaging. *Human Brain Mapping*, 20(3):123–141, 2003.

[9] A. Moelker, R. A. J. J. Maas, and P. M. T. Pattynama. Verbal communication in MR environments: Effect of MR system acoustic noise on speech understanding. *Radiology*, 232(1):107–113, 2004.

[10] K. J. Lasota, J. L. Ulmer, J. B. Firszt, B. B. Biswal, D. L. Daniels, and R. W. Prost. Intensity-dependent activation of the primary auditory cortex in functional magnetic resonance imaging. *Journal of Computer Assisted Tomography*, 27(2):213–218, 2003.

Bibliography

[11] C. J. Scarff, J. C. Dort, J. J. Eggermont, and B. G. Goodyear. The effect of MR scanner noise on auditory cortex activity using fMRI. *Human Brain Mapping*, 22: 341–349, 2004.

[12] D. R. M. Langers, P. van Dijk, and W. H. Backes. Interactions between hemodynamic responses to scanner acoustic noise and auditory stimuli in functional magnetic resonance imaging. *Magnetic Resonance in Medicine*, 53(1):49–60, 2005.

[13] D. Tomasi, E. C. Caparelli, L. Chang, and T. Ernst. fMRI-acoustic noise alters brain activation during working memory tasks. *NeuroImage*, 27:377–386, 2005.

[14] Z. H. Cho, S. C. Chung, D. W. Lim, and E. K. Wong. Effects of the acoustic noise of the gradient systems on fMRI: a study on auditory, motor, and visual cortices. *Magnetic Resonance in Medicine*, 39:331–335, 1998.

[15] N. Zhang, X. H. Zhu, and W. Chen. Influence of gradient acoustic noise on fMRI response in the human visual cortex. *Magnetic Resonance in Medicine*, 54(2):258–263, 2005.

[16] S. Watkins, L. Shams, S. Tanaka, J.-D. Haynes, and G. Rees. Sound alters activity in human V1 in association with illusory visual perception. *NeuroImage*, 31(3): 1247–1256, 2006.

[17] Y. Boyle, D. E. Bentley, A. Watson, and A. K. P. Jones. Acoustic noise in functional magnetic resonance imaging reduces pain unpleasantness ratings. *NeuroImage*, 31 (3):1278–1283, 2006.

[18] P. Mansfield, P. M. Glover, and J. Beaumont. Sound generation in gradient coil structures for MRI. *Magnetic Resonance in Medicine*, 39:539–550, 1998.

[19] P. Mansfield and B. Haywood. Principles of active acoustic control in gradient coil design. *Magnetic Resonance Materials in Physics, Biology and Medicine*, 8(Suppl 1):55, 1999.

[20] P. Mansfield and B. Haywood. Principles of active acoustic control in gradient coil design. *Magnetic Resonance Materials in Physics, Biology and Medicine*, 10: 147–151, 2000.

Bibliography

[21] A. D. Yeo. Quiet magnetic resonance imaging gradients. Master's thesis, University of Queensland, Australia, 2000.

[22] P. Mansfield, B. Haywood, and R. Coxon. Active acoustic control in gradient coils for MRI. *Magnetic Resonance in Medicine*, 46:807–818, 2001.

[23] T. Yoshida, H. Takamori, and A. Katsunuma. EXCELART MRI system with revolutionary pianissimo noise-reduction technology. Technical report, Toshiba, 2000.

[24] A. Katsunuma, H. Takamori, Y. Sakakura, Y. Hamamura, Y. Ogo, and R. Katayama. Quite MRI with novel acoustic noise reduction. *Magnetic Resonance Materials in Physics, Biology and Medicine*, 13:139–144, 2002.

[25] A. Moelker, M. W. Vogel, and P. M. T. Pattynama. Efficacy of passive acoustic screening: Implications for the design of imager and MR-suite. *Journal of Magnetic Resonance Imaging*, 17:270–275, 2003.

[26] W. A. Edelstein, T. K. Kidane, V. Taracila, T. N. Baig, T. P. Eagan, Y. C. N-Cheng, R. W. Brown, and J. A. Mallick. Active-passive gradient shielding for MRI acoustic noise reduction. *Magnetic Resonance in Medicine*, 53(5):1013–1017, 2005.

[27] J. B. Evans. Sound isolation design for a magnetic resonance imaging system (MRI). In *Eleventh International Congress on Sound and Vibration*, pages 591–598, 2004.

[28] K. Liener, A. Wunderlich, G. Ehret, and E. Bachor. Messungen zum Lärmschutz bei der funktionellen MR-Tomographie. *Laryngo-Rhino-Otologie*, 84:108–112, 2005.

[29] M. E. Ravicz and J. R. Melcher. Isolating the auditory system from acoustic noise during functional magnetic resonance imaging: Examination of noise conduction through the ear canal, head, and body. *Journal of the Acoustical Society of America*, 109(1):216–231, 2001.

[30] A. Moelker, R. A. J. J. Maas, M. W. Vogel, M. Ouhlous, and P. M. T. Pattynama. Importance of bone-conducted sound transmission on patient hearing in the MR scanner. *Journal of Magnetic Resonance Imaging*, 22:163–169, 2005.

[31] C. K. Chen, T. D. Chiueh, and J. H. Chen. Active cancellation system of acoustic noise in MR imaging. *IEEE Transactions on Biomedical Engineering*, 46(2):186–191, 1999.

[32] J. Chambers, M. A. Akeroyd, A. Q. Summerfield, and A. R. Palmer. Active control of the volume acquisition noise in functional magnetic resonance imaging: Method and psychoacoustical evaluation. *Journal of the Acoustical Society of America*, 110(6):3041–3054, 2001.

[33] R. Cusack, N. Cumming, D. Bor, D. Norris, and J. Lyzenga. Automated post-hoc noise cancellation tool for audio recordings acquired in an MRI scanner. *Human Brain Mapping*, 24:299–304, 2005.

[34] D. Tomasi and T. Ernst. A simple theory for vibration of MRI gradient coils. *Brazilian Journal of Physics*, 36(1A):34–39, 2006.

[35] T. P. Eagan, T. Baig, J. J. Derakhshan, J. L. Duerk, and R. Brown. Acoustic noise suppression: Gradient self-help? In *Proc. Intl. Soc. Mag. Reson. Med 15*, page 1101, 2007.

[36] X. Chen, X. Shou, T. P. Eagan, and T. W. Brown. Understanding acoustic noise suppression with gradient design: A vibrating string model. In *Proc. Intl. Soc. Mag. Reson. Med 16*, page 2988, 2008.

[37] D. A. Hall, M. P. Haggard, M. A. Akeroyd, A. R. Palmer, A. Q. Summerfield, M. R. Elliot, E. M. Gurney, and R. W. Bowtell. "Sparse" temporal sampling in auditory fMRI. *Human Brain Mapping*, 7:213–223, 1999.

[38] Y. Yang, A. Engelien, W. Engelien, S. Xu, E. Stern, and D. A. Silbersweig. A silent event-related functional MRI technique for brain activation studies without interference of scanner acoustic noise. *Magnetic Resonance in Medicine*, 43(2):185–190, 2000.

[39] J. A. de Zwart, P. van Gelderen, P. Kellman, and J. H. Duyn. Reduction of gradient acoustic noise in MRI using SENSE-EPI. *NeuroImage*, 16:1151–1155, 2002.

[40] F. Hennel, F. Girard, and T. Loenneker. "Silent" MRI with soft gradient pulses. *Magnetic Resonance in Medicine*, 42(1):6–10, 1999.

[41] F. Hennel. Fast spin echo and fast gradient echo MRI with low acoustic noise. *Journal of Magnetic Resonance Imaging*, 13(6):960–966, 2001.

[42] P. Latta, M. L. H. Gruwel, E. Edie, M. Srámek, and B. Tomanek. Single point imaging with suppressed sound pressure levels through gradient-shape adjustment. *Journal of Magnetic Resonance*, 170:177–183, 2004.

[43] J. I. Jackson, C. H. Meyer, D. G. Nishimura, and A. Macovski. Selection of a convolution function for fourier inversion using gridding [computerised tomography application]. *IEEE Transactions on Medical Imaging*, 10(3):473–478, 1991.

[44] D. J. Schaefer, J. D. Bourland, and J. A. Nyenhuis. Review of patient safety in time-varying gradient fields. *Journal of Magnetic Resonance Imaging*, 12(1):20–29, 2000.

[45] D. G. Tomasi and T. Ernst. Echo planar imaging at 4 Tesla with minimum acoustic noise. *Journal of Magnetic Resonance Imaging*, 18:128–130, 2003.

[46] E. Seifritz, F. Di Salle, F. Esposito, M. Herdener, J. G. Neuhoff, and K. Scheffler. Enhancing BOLD response in the auditory system by neurophysiologically tuned fMRI sequence. *NeuroImage*, 29:1013–1022, 2006.

[47] S. Schmitter. *Entwicklung von geräuscharmen Bildgebungstechniken für die funktionelle Magnetresonanztomographie*. PhD thesis, Universität Heidelberg, 2008.

[48] F. Kameier and D. Reinartz. Strömungsakustik. Seminar, Fachhochschule Düsseldorf, 2001.

6. Summary

6.1. Conclusion

The Hilbert-Moore sequence is the first gradient echo imaging sequence built from scratch with acoustic noise reduction being the major concern. In conventional approaches it is tried to attenuate the acoustic noise generated by a pulse sequence by modification of the gradient waveform or the scanner hardware. In contrast to the conventional approaches, the Hilbert-Moore sequence tries to exploit the generation mechanism of the acoustic noise during MR image acquisition. The acoustic noise is generated by the switching of the encoding gradients. The basic idea of the Hilbert-Moore sequence is to apply a very frequent, feigned stochastic gradient switching on both gradient encoding axis and thus shift the major sound energy generated by the gradients possibly above the human hearing threshold.

Due to hardware limitations like the gradient's slewrate and the gradient raster time acoustic noise is still audible during the execution of the Hilbert-Moore imaging sequence. However, a broader distribution of the sound energy over the complete hearing range, in addition with a shift of the major sound energy to higher frequencies has been achieved. Conventional pulse sequences like EPI emit their peak sound energy in a frequency range from 500Hz to 1500Hz which is the bandwidth of the human phonation. The Hilbert-Moore sequence shifted the peak sound energy to frequencies above 4000Hz which allows for better damping by conventional means like ear plugs. In addition, the broader frequency distribution of the acoustic noise emitted by the Hilbert-Moore sequence leads to a smoother sound characteristic which is more favorable for the human hearing system than the hard pulsed sounds emitted by a standard EPI sequence.

The speciality of the Hilbert-Moore sequence is the direct addressing of adjacent neighbors along the Hilbert-Moore space filling curve. Moving from one k-space point to a directly adjacent one requires only a small gradient amplitude applied during a short

6. Summary

time. In the Hilbert-Moore sequence every step from one k-space point to an adjacent one is realized by a triangular gradient blip. It has been shown that the short small amplitude triangular gradient blips used in the Hilbert-Moore sequence are not liable to eddy current influences. So the designed trajectory is followed with scarce aberrations only.

The image quality of the Hilbert-Moore sequence proved to be acceptable for a resolution of 64 × 64 k-space points. The equable distribution of the gradient load on both gradient axis reduces the geometric distortions present in other sequences with an uneven distribution of the gradient load, like EPI for example. The twofold undersampling in both gradient directions leads to a widespread, steady distribution of the artifacts introduced by the undersampling. Leaving k-space lines empty in an EPI sequence leads to ghosting artifacts. The object to be imaged appears at different fixed positions in the image with different intensities. In the Hilbert-Moore sequence the twofold undersampling leads to a distribution of the resulting artifacts all over the image and thus, to an increase of the background noise.

Overall, the Hilbert-Moore sequence is a quite promising approach and could be a predecessor of a new class of imaging sequences designed for the reduction of acoustic noise during MR image acquisition.

6.2. Outlook

The full potential of the Hilbert-Moore sequence has not yet been reached. A variety of improvements concerning sound noise emittance and image quality are possible.

The herein presented proof-of-principle uses a conventional, trapezoidal slice selection gradient. For the sound measurements the flip angle has been restricted to 5° resulting also in low influence of the slice selection gradient. By switching off the slice selection gradient (and the RF pulse) a reduction of the sound pressure level about 1dB is achieved. For larger flip angles (e.g. 90°) the contribution of the slice selection gradient is clearly audible during execution of the sequence. By adjusting the slice selection gradient to e.g. a sinusoidal instead of a trapezoidal waveform or by other means a further reduction of the acoustic noise generated by the Hilbert-Moore sequence should be possible.

The restriction to 64 × 64 pixels is today's standard for fMRI images with an EPI sequence but a higher resolution is desirable. Improvement of the image resolution can be achieved by two means. By adjusting the gradient blip size so that instead of covering two Δk steps with each blip a larger number of Δk steps is covered (e.g. 4) higher resolutions of e.g. 128×128 could be realized easily. However, a doubling in the execution time for each blip leads to a doubling of the total execution time of the sequence. It has to be evaluated if the execution of the sequence can then be realized fast enough to acquire a sufficient signal strength for every sampled k-space point if signal decay is taken into account. Furthermore, it has to be evaluated if the developed reconstruction algorithm still holds for the new neighborhood relations generated by this approach.

The second option is multishot imaging. With each RF excitation (shot) a 64×64 matrix could be acquired and by combining the acquired matrices a larger k-space matrix could be realized. An image with a resolution of 128×128 could be realized by two shots if inherent k-space symmetry is exploited to select the 64×64 sub-matrices. Disadvantages of the multishot approach are the increased total imaging time, the higher RF load and the difficulty to match the borders of the acquired sub-matrices. Especially motion or a slightly changed position of the subject during the acquisition of the individual parts are a prominent source of errors.

To improve the image quality of the Hilbert-Moore an enhancement of the reconstruction algorithm is imaginable. The reconstruction algorithm presented herein calculated a missing point out of a single direct neighbor. By including multiple neighbors in the reconstruction of a missing point, the stability of the reconstruction algorithm should improve and its susceptibility to outliers is expected to reduce. However, including multiple points in the reconstruction leads to more complex neighborhood patterns to be found in the image and larger matrices have to be inverted during the weighting calculation. So a higher computational load is to be expected.

Another possibility to improve the overall image quality of the Hilbert-Moore sequence is the correction of the signal decay due to relaxation effects. For the Hilbert-Moore sequence, the exact sampling time point for every point in k-space is known due to the individual addressing of k-space points along the Hilbert-Moore space filling curve. Thus, the corresponding signal decay could be calculated for each sampled point and the acquired signal could be amplified, revoking the signal decay. The difficulty in this approach is that usually not a single material with fixed relaxation constants is present in the sample. For a more complex sample (like a human being or an animal) a variety of materials having different relaxation constants are present and contribute

6. Summary

to the signal. So for each single spin, the effect of the gradients and the signal decay has to be computed. For the Hilbert-Moore sequence one k-space point corresponds to a volume of $3.9 \times 3.9 \times 2mm$ for a FOV of 250mm and a slice thickness of 2mm, it is impossible to compute the correction factor for each k-space point in a reasonable amount of time with the computing power available today.

Ideally, the presented Hilbert-Moore sequence is just the start for a new generation of different pulse sequences optimized for acoustic noise imaging. In contrast to attenuate the acoustic noise generated by the gradient coils, in the new generation of pulse sequences the acoustic noise generation is exploited to reduce the acoustic noise generated during execution of an imaging sequence. Especially the idea of self-helping gradient sequences, which generate the counter wave needed for active noise cancellation by itself, has some potential. One possibility to capitalize on this idea could be to sample k-space along a Lissajous pattern. Launching individual sine-waves on each gradient axes could -by correct adjustment of the phases- lead to a cancellation of the sound energy generated during execution. Difficulties of this approach would be the correct adjustment of the phase of the sine waves and once again the execution time of the sequence. In addition, the non-cartesian sampling along a Lissajous pattern would lead to a large computational effort for the reconstruction algorithm.

A. Gradient encoding tables

A.1. Replacement factors

```
static const long REPLACE_MULT[7]     = {4, 6, 8, 10, 12, 14, 16}; // Length of Stretching Array Entries
static const float REPLACE_FACTS[7][16] = {
  /* 2 GRT Units */
  {0.50, 1.00, 0.50, 0.00, 0.00, 0.00, 0.00, 0.00, 0.00, 0.00, 0.00, 0.00, 0.00, 0.00, 0.00, 0.00},
  /* 3 GRT Units */
  {0.33, 0.67, 1.00, 0.67, 0.33, 0.00, 0.00, 0.00, 0.00, 0.00, 0.00, 0.00, 0.00, 0.00, 0.00, 0.00},
  /* 4 GRT Units */
  {0.25, 0.50, 0.75, 1.00, 0.75, 0.50, 0.25, 0.00, 0.00, 0.00, 0.00, 0.00, 0.00, 0.00, 0.00, 0.00},
  /* 5 GRT Units */
  {0.20, 0.40, 0.60, 0.80, 1.00, 0.80, 0.60, 0.40, 0.20, 0.00, 0.00, 0.00, 0.00, 0.00, 0.00, 0.00},
  /* 6 GRT Units */
  {0.16, 0.33, 0.50, 0.66, 0.82, 1.00, 0.82, 0.66, 0.50, 0.33, 0.16, 0.00, 0.00, 0.00, 0.00, 0.00},
  /* 7 GRT Units */
  {0.14, 0.28, 0.42, 0.57, 0.71, 0.85, 1.00, 0.85, 0.71, 0.57, 0.42, 0.28, 0.14, 0.00, 0.00, 0.00},
  /* 8 GRT Units */
  {0.12, 0.25, 0.37, 0.50, 0.62, 0.75, 0.87, 1.00, 0.87, 0.75, 0.62, 0.50, 0.37, 0.25, 0.12, 0.00}
}; // REPLACE_Facts
```

A.2. Gradient settings for VD center

```
static float GRAD_BLOCK_8x8_X[] = {
  0.0,-1.0, 0.0,-1.0,-1.0, 0.0, 1.0, 0.0,-1.0, 0.0, 1.0, 1.0, 0.0, 1.0, 0.0,
  0.0,
  0.0,-1.0, 0.0,-1.0,-1.0, 0.0, 1.0, 0.0,-1.0, 0.0, 1.0, 1.0, 0.0, 1.0, 0.0,
  1.0,
  0.0, 1.0, 0.0, 1.0, 1.0, 0.0,-1.0, 0.0, 1.0, 0.0,-1.0,-1.0, 0.0,-1.0, 0.0,
  0.0,
  0.0, 1.0, 0.0, 1.0, 1.0, 0.0,-1.0, 0.0, 1.0, 0.0,-1.0,-1.0, 0.0,-1.0, 0.0,
  -1.0
};
static float GRAD_BLOCK_8x8_Y[] = {
  1.0, 0.0,-1.0, 0.0, 0.0, 1.0, 0.0, 1.0, 0.0, 1.0, 0.0, 0.0,-1.0, 0.0, 1.0,
  1.0,
  1.0, 0.0,-1.0, 0.0, 0.0, 1.0, 0.0, 1.0, 0.0, 1.0, 0.0, 0.0,-1.0, 0.0, 1.0,
  0.0,
  -1.0, 0.0, 1.0, 0.0, 0.0,-1.0, 0.0,-1.0, 0.0,-1.0, 0.0, 0.0, 1.0, 0.0,-1.0,
  -1.0,
  -1.0, 0.0, 1.0, 0.0, 0.0,-1.0, 0.0,-1.0, 0.0,-1.0, 0.0, 0.0, 1.0, 0.0,-1.0,
  0.0
};
```

A.3. Gradient settings for HM trajectory

A. Gradient encoding tables

```c
static float GRAD_BLOCK_X[] = {
    0.0,-1.0, 0.0,-1.0,-1.0, 0.0, 1.0, 0.0,-1.0, 0.0, 1.0, 1.0, 0.0, 1.0, 0.0, 0.0,-1.0, 0.0, 1.0, 0.0, 0.0,
   -1.0, 0.0,-1.0, 0.0,-1.0, 0.0, 0.0, 1.0, 0.0, 0.0,-1.0,-1.0, 0.0, 1.0, 0.0, 0.0, 0.0,-1.0, 0.0,-1.0,
    0.0, 0.0, 1.0, 0.0,-1.0, 0.0, 0.0, 1.0, 0.0, 1.0, 1.0, 0.0,-1.0, 0.0, 1.0, 0.0,-1.0,-1.0, 0.0,-1.0, 0.0,
   -1.0,-1.0, 0.0, 1.0, 0.0, 0.0, 0.0,-1.0, 0.0,-1.0, 0.0, 0.0, 1.0, 0.0, 0.0,-1.0,-1.0, 0.0,-1.0, 0.0,-1.0,
   -1.0, 0.0, 1.0, 0.0,-1.0, 0.0, 1.0, 1.0, 0.0, 1.0, 0.0, 0.0, 0.0,-1.0, 0.0,-1.0,-1.0, 0.0, 1.0, 0.0,-1.0,
    0.0, 1.0, 1.0, 0.0, 1.0, 0.0, 1.0, 1.0, 0.0,-1.0, 0.0, 0.0, 1.0, 0.0, 1.0, 0.0, 1.0, 0.0,-1.0, 0.0,
    1.0, 0.0,-1.0, 0.0, 1.0, 0.0, 0.0, 0.0,-1.0, 0.0,-1.0, 0.0, 0.0, 0.0,-1.0, 0.0, 1.0, 0.0,-1.0,-1.0, 0.0,-1.0, 0.0,
   -1.0,-1.0, 0.0, 1.0, 0.0,-1.0, 0.0, 1.0, 1.0, 0.0, 1.0, 0.0, 0.0, 0.0,-1.0, 0.0,-1.0,-1.0, 0.0, 1.0, 0.0,
   -1.0, 0.0, 1.0, 0.0, 1.0, 0.0, 1.0, 1.0, 0.0,-1.0, 0.0, 1.0, 0.0, 0.0, 1.0, 0.0, 1.0, 0.0, 0.0,-1.0, 0.0,
    0.0, 1.0, 1.0, 0.0, 1.0, 0.0, 1.0, 1.0, 0.0,-1.0, 0.0, 1.0, 0.0,-1.0,-1.0, 0.0,-1.0, 0.0, 0.0, 1.0, 0.0,
   -1.0, 0.0, 0.0, 1.0, 0.0, 1.0, 0.0, 1.0, 0.0, 0.0, 1.0, 0.0, 0.0,-1.0, 0.0, 1.0, 1.0, 0.0,-1.0, 0.0, 0.0, 0.0, 1.0, 0.0,
    1.0, 0.0, 1.0, 0.0, 0.0,-1.0, 0.0, 1.0, 0.0, 0.0,-1.0, 0.0,-1.0,-1.0, 0.0, 1.0, 0.0,-1.0, 0.0, 1.0, 1.0,
    0.0, 1.0, 0.0, 0.0, 0.0,-1.0, 0.0,-1.0,-1.0, 0.0, 1.0, 0.0,-1.0, 0.0, 1.0, 1.0, 0.0, 1.0, 0.0, 0.0,-1.0,
    0.0, 1.0, 0.0, 0.0,-1.0, 0.0,-1.0, 0.0, 0.0, 1.0, 0.0,-1.0,-1.0,-1.0, 0.0, 1.0, 0.0, 0.0,-1.0,
    0.0,-1.0, 0.0,-1.0, 0.0, 0.0, 1.0, 0.0,-1.0, 0.0, 0.0, 1.0, 0.0, 1.0, 1.0, 0.0,-1.0, 0.0, 1.0, 0.0,-1.0,
   -1.0, 0.0,-1.0, 0.0,-1.0,-1.0, 0.0, 1.0, 0.0, 0.0,-1.0, 0.0,-1.0, 0.0, 0.0,-1.0, 0.0, 0.0, 1.0, 0.0,-1.0,-1.0,
    0.0,-1.0, 0.0,-1.0,-1.0, 0.0, 1.0, 0.0,-1.0, 0.0, 1.0, 1.0, 0.0, 0.0, 0.0,-1.0, 0.0,-1.0, 0.0,
    0.0, 1.0, 0.0,-1.0, 0.0, 1.0, 1.0, 0.0, 1.0, 0.0, 1.0, 1.0, 0.0,-1.0, 0.0, 0.0, 1.0, 0.0, 0.0, 1.0, 1.0,
    0.0, 0.0,-1.0, 0.0, 1.0, 0.0,-1.0, 0.0, 1.0, 0.0, 0.0,-1.0, 0.0,-1.0, 0.0, 0.0,-1.0, 0.0, 0.0, 1.0, 0.0,
   -1.0, 0.0,-1.0, 0.0,-1.0,-1.0, 0.0, 1.0, 0.0,-1.0, 0.0, 1.0, 1.0, 0.0, 1.0, 0.0, 0.0, 0.0,-1.0, 0.0,-1.0,
   -1.0, 0.0, 1.0, 0.0,-1.0, 0.0, 1.0, 1.0, 0.0, 1.0, 0.0, 1.0, 1.0, 0.0,-1.0, 0.0, 0.0, 1.0, 0.0, 1.0, 0.0,
    1.0, 0.0, 0.0,-1.0, 0.0, 1.0, 0.0, 1.0, 0.0, 0.0, 1.0, 0.0, 1.0, 0.0,-1.0, 0.0, 1.0, 0.0,-1.0,-1.0, 0.0,-1.0,
    0.0, 0.0, 1.0, 0.0,-1.0, 0.0, 0.0, 1.0, 0.0, 1.0, 0.0, 0.0, 0.0,-1.0, 0.0, 0.0,-1.0, 0.0, 1.0, 0.0,
   -1.0, 0.0, 1.0, 1.0, 0.0, 1.0, 0.0, 1.0, 0.0, 1.0, 1.0, 0.0,-1.0, 0.0, 0.0, 0.0,-1.0,-1.0, 0.0, 0.0,
   -1.0, 0.0, 0.0, 1.0, 0.0,-1.0, 0.0, 0.0, 1.0, 0.0, 1.0, 0.0, 0.0, 0.0,-1.0, 0.0, 1.0, 1.0, 1.0, 0.0,
   -1.0, 0.0, 0.0, 1.0, 0.0, 1.0, 0.0, 1.0, 0.0, 0.0,-1.0, 0.0, 1.0, 0.0, 0.0,-1.0, 0.0,-1.0,-1.0, 0.0, 1.0,
    0.0,-1.0, 0.0, 1.0, 1.0, 0.0, 1.0, 0.0, 1.0, 1.0, 0.0,-1.0, 0.0, 0.0, 1.0, 0.0, 1.0, 0.0, 1.0, 0.0, 0.0,
   -1.0, 0.0, 1.0, 1.0, 0.0, 1.0, 0.0, 1.0, 1.0, 0.0,-1.0, 0.0, 1.0, 0.0,-1.0,-1.0, 0.0,-1.0, 0.0, 0.0, 0.0,
    1.0, 0.0, 1.0, 1.0, 0.0,-1.0, 0.0, 1.0, 0.0,-1.0,-1.0, 0.0, 1.0, 0.0,-1.0,-1.0, 0.0, 1.0, 0.0, 0.0,-1.0,
    0.0,-1.0, 0.0,-1.0, 0.0, 0.0, 1.0, 0.0,-1.0, 0.0, 0.0, 1.0, 0.0,-1.0, 0.0, 0.0, 1.0, 0.0, 1.0, 0.0, 1.0, 0.0,
    0.0,-1.0, 0.0, 0.0, 1.0, 1.0, 0.0, 1.0, 0.0, 1.0, 1.0, 0.0,-1.0,-1.0, 0.0,-1.0, 0.0,-1.0,-1.0, 0.0,-1.0, 0.0,
    0.0, 1.0, 0.0, 0.0, 1.0, 0.0,-1.0, 0.0, 1.0, 0.0,-1.0,-1.0, 0.0,-1.0, 0.0,-1.0,-1.0, 0.0, 1.0, 0.0, 0.0,
   -1.0, 0.0,-1.0, 0.0,-1.0,-1.0, 0.0, 1.0, 0.0,-1.0,-1.0, 0.0,-1.0, 0.0, 0.0, 0.0, 1.0, 0.0,-1.0, 0.0, 0.0, 0.0,
    1.0, 0.0, 0.0,-1.0, 0.0, 1.0, 0.0,-1.0,-1.0, 0.0,-1.0, 0.0, 0.0,-1.0, 0.0, 0.0, 1.0, 0.0,-1.0, 0.0, 0.0, 1.0,
   -1.0,-1.0, 0.0, 1.0, 0.0, 0.0,-1.0, 0.0,-1.0, 0.0,-1.0, 0.0, 0.0, 0.0, 1.0, 0.0,-1.0, 0.0, 0.0, 0.0, 1.0, 0.0, 1.0,
    1.0, 0.0,-1.0, 0.0, 1.0, 0.0,-1.0,-1.0, 0.0,-1.0, 0.0, 0.0, 1.0, 0.0, 1.0, 1.0, 0.0,-1.0, 0.0, 0.0, 1.0,
    0.0,-1.0,-1.0, 0.0,-1.0, 0.0, 0.0, 1.0, 0.0,-1.0, 0.0, 0.0, 1.0, 0.0, 1.0, 0.0, 1.0, 0.0, 0.0,-1.0, 0.0,
    1.0, 1.0, 0.0,-1.0, 0.0, 0.0, 1.0, 0.0, 1.0, 1.0, 0.0,-1.0, 0.0, 1.0, 0.0, 1.0, 1.0, 0.0, 0.0,-1.0, 0.0, 0.0,
   -1.0,-1.0, 0.0, 1.0, 0.0,-1.0, 0.0, 1.0, 1.0, 0.0, 1.0, 0.0, 1.0, 1.0, 0.0,-1.0,-1.0, 0.0, 1.0, 0.0, 1.0,
    0.0, 1.0, 0.0, 0.0, 0.0, 1.0, 0.0, 1.0, 1.0, 0.0,-1.0, 0.0, 1.0, 0.0,-1.0,-1.0, 0.0,-1.0,-1.0, 0.0, 0.0,
    1.0, 0.0, 0.0,-1.0, 0.0,-1.0, 0.0,-1.0, 0.0, 0.0, 1.0, 0.0,-1.0, 0.0, 0.0, 1.0, 0.0,-1.0, 0.0, 0.0, 1.0, 0.0,
    1.0, 0.0, 1.0, 1.0, 0.0,-1.0, 0.0,-1.0, 0.0, 0.0, 1.0, 0.0,-1.0, 0.0, 0.0, 1.0, 1.0, 0.0,-1.0,-1.0, 0.0,-1.0,-1.0,
    0.0, 1.0, 0.0, 0.0,-1.0, 0.0,-1.0, 0.0, 0.0, 0.0,-1.0, 0.0,-1.0, 0.0, 0.0, 1.0, 0.0,-1.0,-1.0, 0.0,-1.0, 0.0,
    1.0, 0.0,-1.0, 0.0, 1.0, 0.0, 1.0, 0.0, 0.0, 0.0,-1.0, 0.0, 1.0, 0.0, 0.0,-1.0, 0.0,-1.0, 0.0,-1.0, 0.0,
    0.0, 1.0, 0.0,-1.0,-1.0,-1.0, 0.0, 1.0, 0.0, 0.0,-1.0, 0.0,-1.0, 0.0, 0.0,-1.0, 0.0, 0.0, 1.0, 0.0,-1.0, 0.0, 0.0,
    0.0, 1.0, 0.0, 1.0, 1.0, 0.0,-1.0, 0.0, 1.0, 0.0,-1.0,-1.0, 0.0,-1.0, 0.0, 0.0,-1.0
}; // GRAD_BLOCK_X

static float GRAD_BLOCK_Y[] = {
    1.0, 0.0,-1.0, 0.0, 0.0, 1.0, 0.0, 0.0, 1.0, 0.0, 0.0,-1.0, 0.0, 0.0, 1.0, 0.0, 1.0, 0.0, 0.0, 1.0, 1.0,
    0.0,-1.0, 0.0, 1.0, 0.0,-1.0,-1.0, 0.0,-1.0, 0.0, 0.0, 0.0, 1.0, 0.0, 1.0, 1.0, 0.0,-1.0, 0.0, 1.0, 0.0,
   -1.0,-1.0, 0.0,-1.0, 0.0, 0.0, 1.0, 0.0, 0.0,-1.0, 0.0,-1.0, 0.0,-1.0, 0.0, 0.0, 0.0, 1.0, 0.0,-1.0, 0.0,
    0.0, 0.0, 1.0, 0.0, 1.0, 1.0, 0.0,-1.0, 0.0, 1.0, 0.0,-1.0,-1.0, 0.0,-1.0, 0.0, 0.0, 1.0, 0.0,-1.0, 0.0,
    0.0, 1.0, 0.0, 1.0, 0.0, 1.0, 0.0, 0.0,-1.0, 0.0, 1.0, 1.0, 1.0, 0.0,-1.0, 0.0, 0.0, 1.0, 0.0, 1.0, 0.0,
    1.0, 0.0, 0.0,-1.0, 0.0, 1.0, 0.0, 0.0,-1.0,-1.0, 0.0, 0.0, 1.0, 0.0, 0.0, 1.0, 0.0, 1.0, 0.0, 1.0, 0.0,
    0.0, 1.0, 0.0, 1.0, 0.0, 1.0, 1.0, 0.0,-1.0, 0.0, 1.0, 0.0,-1.0,-1.0, 0.0,-1.0, 0.0, 0.0, 1.0, 0.0,-1.0,
    0.0, 1.0, 0.0, 0.0,-1.0, 0.0, 1.0, 0.0, 0.0,-1.0, 0.0,-1.0,-1.0, 0.0, 1.0, 0.0,-1.0, 0.0, 1.0, 0.0, 0.0,
    1.0, 0.0, 0.0,-1.0, 0.0, 1.0, 0.0, 0.0,-1.0, 0.0,-1.0,-1.0, 0.0, 0.0, 0.0, 0.0, 1.0, 0.0,-1.0, 0.0, 0.0,-1.0,
    0.0,-1.0,-1.0, 0.0, 1.0, 0.0,-1.0, 0.0, 1.0, 1.0, 0.0, 1.0, 0.0, 0.0, 0.0,-1.0, 0.0,-1.0,-1.0, 0.0,-1.0,
    0.0,-1.0, 0.0, 1.0, 1.0, 0.0, 1.0, 0.0, 1.0, 1.0, 0.0,-1.0, 0.0, 0.0, 1.0, 0.0, 1.0, 0.0, 1.0, 0.0, 0.0,
   -1.0, 0.0, 1.0, 1.0, 0.0,-1.0, 0.0, 0.0, 0.0, 1.0, 0.0, 1.0, 0.0, 0.0,-1.0, 0.0, 1.0, 0.0, 0.0, 1.0,
    1.0, 0.0, 1.0, 1.0, 0.0,-1.0, 0.0, 1.0, 0.0,-1.0,-1.0, 0.0,-1.0, 0.0, 0.0, 0.0, 1.0, 0.0, 1.0, 0.0, 1.0,
   -1.0, 0.0, 1.0, 0.0,-1.0,-1.0, 0.0,-1.0, 0.0,-1.0,-1.0, 0.0, 1.0, 0.0, 0.0,-1.0, 0.0,-1.0, 0.0,-1.0, 0.0,
    0.0, 1.0, 0.0,-1.0, 0.0, 0.0, 1.0, 0.0, 1.0, 1.0, 0.0,-1.0, 0.0, 1.0, 0.0,-1.0,-1.0, 0.0,-1.0, 0.0, 0.0,
```

100

A. Gradient encoding tables

```
    1.0, 0.0,-1.0, 0.0, 0.0, 1.0, 0.0, 1.0, 0.0, 1.0, 0.0, 0.0,-1.0, 0.0, 1.0, 1.0, 1.0, 0.0,-1.0, 0.0, 0.0,
    1.0, 0.0, 1.0, 0.0, 1.0, 0.0, 0.0,-1.0, 0.0, 1.0, 0.0, 0.0,-1.0, 0.0,-1.0,-1.0, 0.0, 1.0, 0.0,-1.0, 0.0,
    1.0, 1.0, 0.0, 1.0, 0.0, 0.0, 1.0, 0.0, 1.0, 1.0, 0.0,-1.0, 0.0, 1.0, 0.0,-1.0,-1.0, 0.0,-1.0, 0.0,
    0.0, 1.0, 0.0,-1.0, 0.0, 0.0, 1.0, 0.0, 1.0, 0.0, 1.0, 0.0, 0.0,-1.0, 0.0, 1.0, 1.0, 1.0, 0.0,-1.0, 0.0,
    0.0, 1.0, 0.0, 1.0, 0.0, 1.0, 0.0, 0.0,-1.0, 0.0, 1.0, 0.0, 0.0,-1.0, 0.0,-1.0,-1.0, 0.0, 1.0, 0.0,-1.0,
    0.0, 1.0, 1.0, 0.0, 1.0, 0.0, 0.0,-1.0, 0.0, 1.0, 0.0, 0.0,-1.0, 0.0,-1.0, 0.0,-1.0, 0.0, 0.0, 1.0, 0.0,
   -1.0,-1.0, 0.0,-1.0, 0.0,-1.0,-1.0, 0.0, 1.0, 0.0,-1.0, 0.0, 1.0, 1.0, 0.0, 1.0, 0.0, 0.0, 0.0,-1.0, 0.0,
   -1.0,-1.0, 0.0, 1.0, 0.0,-1.0, 0.0, 1.0, 1.0, 0.0, 1.0, 0.0, 1.0, 1.0, 0.0,-1.0, 0.0, 0.0, 1.0, 0.0, 1.0,
    0.0, 1.0, 0.0, 0.0,-1.0, 0.0, 1.0, 0.0,-1.0, 0.0, 1.0, 0.0, 0.0,-1.0, 0.0,-1.0, 0.0,-1.0, 0.0, 0.0, 1.0,
    0.0,-1.0,-1.0, 0.0,-1.0, 0.0,-1.0,-1.0, 0.0, 1.0, 0.0,-1.0, 0.0, 1.0, 1.0, 0.0, 1.0, 0.0, 0.0, 0.0,-1.0,
    0.0,-1.0,-1.0, 0.0, 1.0, 0.0,-1.0, 0.0, 1.0, 1.0, 0.0, 1.0, 0.0, 1.0, 1.0, 0.0,-1.0, 0.0, 0.0, 1.0, 0.0,
    1.0, 0.0, 1.0, 0.0, 0.0,-1.0, 0.0, 1.0, 0.0, 0.0,-1.0, 0.0,-1.0,-1.0, 0.0, 1.0, 0.0,-1.0, 0.0, 1.0, 1.0,
    0.0, 1.0, 0.0, 0.0,-1.0, 0.0, 1.0, 0.0, 0.0,-1.0, 0.0,-1.0, 0.0,-1.0, 0.0, 0.0, 1.0, 0.0,-1.0,-1.0,-1.0,
    0.0, 1.0, 0.0, 0.0,-1.0, 0.0,-1.0, 0.0,-1.0, 0.0, 0.0, 1.0, 0.0,-1.0, 0.0, 0.0, 1.0, 0.0, 1.0, 0.0,
   -1.0, 0.0, 1.0, 0.0,-1.0,-1.0, 0.0,-1.0, 0.0,-1.0, 0.0,-1.0, 0.0,-1.0,-1.0, 0.0, 1.0, 0.0,-1.0, 0.0, 1.0,
    1.0, 0.0, 1.0, 0.0, 0.0,-1.0, 0.0, 1.0, 0.0, 0.0,-1.0, 0.0,-1.0, 0.0,-1.0, 0.0, 0.0, 1.0, 0.0,-1.0,-1.0,
   -1.0, 0.0, 1.0, 0.0, 0.0,-1.0, 0.0,-1.0, 0.0,-1.0,-1.0, 0.0, 0.0, 1.0, 0.0,-1.0, 0.0, 0.0, 1.0, 0.0, 1.0,
    0.0,-1.0, 0.0, 1.0, 0.0,-1.0,-1.0, 0.0,-1.0, 0.0, 0.0, 1.0, 0.0,-1.0, 0.0, 0.0, 1.0, 0.0, 1.0, 0.0, 1.0,
    0.0, 0.0,-1.0, 0.0, 1.0, 1.0, 0.0, 1.0, 0.0, 1.0, 0.0,-1.0, 0.0, 0.0, 1.0, 0.0,-1.0,-1.0, 0.0,-1.0, 0.0,
    0.0, 0.0, 1.0, 0.0, 1.0, 1.0, 0.0,-1.0, 0.0, 1.0, 0.0,-1.0,-1.0, 0.0,-1.0,-1.0, 0.0, 1.0, 0.0,
    0.0,-1.0, 0.0,-1.0, 0.0,-1.0, 0.0, 0.0, 1.0, 0.0,-1.0,-1.0,-1.0, 0.0, 1.0, 0.0, 0.0, 0.0,-1.0, 0.0,
   -1.0, 0.0, 0.0, 1.0, 0.0,-1.0,-1.0, 0.0,-1.0, 0.0,-1.0,-1.0, 0.0, 1.0, 0.0,-1.0, 0.0, 1.0, 1.0, 0.0, 1.0,
    0.0, 0.0, 0.0,-1.0, 0.0,-1.0,-1.0, 0.0,-1.0, 0.0, 1.0, 0.0, 0.0,-1.0, 0.0, 1.0, 0.0, 1.0, 0.0, 1.0, 0.0,
    0.0, 0.0, 1.0, 0.0, 1.0, 0.0, 1.0, 0.0, 0.0,-1.0, 0.0, 1.0, 0.0, 0.0,-1.0, 0.0,-1.0,-1.0, 0.0, 1.0, 0.0,
   -1.0, 0.0, 1.0, 1.0, 0.0, 1.0, 0.0, 0.0,-1.0, 0.0, 1.0, 0.0, 0.0,-1.0, 0.0,-1.0, 0.0,-1.0, 0.0, 0.0, 1.0,
    0.0,-1.0,-1.0,-1.0, 0.0, 1.0, 0.0, 0.0,-1.0, 0.0,-1.0, 0.0, 0.0, 1.0, 0.0,-1.0, 0.0, 0.0, 1.0,
    0.0,-1.0, 0.0, 1.0, 0.0, 0.0, 1.0, 0.0,-1.0, 0.0, 1.0, 0.0, 0.0,-1.0, 0.0,-1.0, 0.0,-1.0, 0.0, 0.0, 1.0,
    1.0, 0.0,-1.0,-1.0,-1.0, 0.0, 1.0, 0.0, 0.0,-1.0, 0.0,-1.0, 0.0,-1.0, 0.0, 0.0, 1.0, 0.0,-1.0, 0.0, 0.0,
    1.0, 0.0, 1.0, 0.0, 0.0,-1.0, 0.0, 1.0, 0.0,-1.0,-1.0, 0.0,-1.0, 0.0, 0.0, 1.0, 0.0, 1.0, 0.0, 0.0, 1.0,
    0.0, 1.0, 0.0, 1.0, 0.0, 0.0,-1.0, 0.0, 1.0, 1.0, 0.0, 1.0, 0.0, 1.0, 1.0, 0.0,-1.0, 0.0, 0.0, 1.0, 0.0,-1.0,
   -1.0, 0.0,-1.0, 0.0, 0.0, 0.0, 1.0, 0.0, 1.0, 1.0, 0.0,-1.0, 0.0, 1.0, 0.0,-1.0,-1.0, 0.0,-1.0, 0.0,-1.0,
   -1.0, 0.0, 1.0, 0.0, 0.0,-1.0, 0.0,-1.0, 0.0,-1.0, 0.0, 0.0, 1.0, 0.0,-1.0, 0.0
}; // GRAD_BLOCK_Y
```

B. Calibration Sound Pressure Levels

B. Calibration Sound Pressure Levels

Table B.1.: *Calibration Tunes Lookup Table connecting Amplitude to Sound Pressure Level for the Octave Band Middle frequencies*

dB	125Hz	250Hz	500Hz	1000Hz	2000Hz	3000Hz	4000Hz	6000Hz	8000Hz	10000Hz
49					1,302	0,325	0,301			
50				5,940	1,586	0,386	0,358	4,231		0,705
51				6,837	1,844	0,442	0,410	5,177	3,157	0,780
52				7,726	2,084	0,495	0,460	6,030	3,919	0,864
53			9,742	8,642	2,317	0,547	0,509	6,822	4,590	0,961
54			12,634	9,621	2,551	0,600	0,559	7,586	5,199	1,072
55			15,033	10,696	2,797	0,656	0,612	8,352	5,771	1,201
56			17,047	11,903	3,064	0,718	0,671	9,154	6,333	1,350
57			18,784	13,277	3,363	0,788	0,737	10,024	6,912	1,521
58			20,354	14,852	3,701	0,867	0,812	10,994	7,532	1,717
59		33,239	21,865	16,664	4,090	0,959	0,898	12,096	8,222	1,940
60		41,799	23,425	18,747	4,539	1,065	0,998	13,362	9,006	2,193
61		49,271	25,142	21,130	5,058	1,188	1,113	14,825	9,912	2,479
62		55,957	27,126	23,820	5,656	1,329	1,246	16,517	10,967	2,800
63		62,156	29,484	26,817	6,343	1,492	1,397	18,470	12,195	3,159
64		68,172	32,326	30,123	7,128	1,677	1,570	20,716	13,624	3,557
65		74,305	35,759	33,738	8,022	1,888	1,767	23,288	15,280	3,998
66	201,265	80,856	39,892	37,683	9,034	2,126	1,989	26,217	17,189	4,484
67	202,991	88,126	44,835	42,063	10,173	2,394	2,238	29,536	19,378	5,018
68	213,956	96,417	50,694	47,003	11,450	2,693	2,516	33,277	21,873	5,601
69	234,160	106,030	57,579	52,627	12,874	3,027	2,826	37,472	24,700	6,238
70	263,601	117,267	65,598	59,060	14,458	3,398	3,170	42,154	27,886	6,929
71	302,280	130,427	74,860	66,412	16,233	3,811	3,555	47,365	31,458	7,680
72	350,198	145,814	85,473	74,726	18,233	4,274	3,987	53,184	35,442	8,503
73	407,354	163,728	97,546	84,032	20,493	4,792	4,473	59,703	39,871	9,412
74	473,748	184,470	111,188	94,358	23,046	5,373	5,020	67,012	44,781	10,422
75	549,380	208,341	126,516	105,733	25,922	6,023	5,635	75,202	50,205	11,546
76	634,250	235,643	143,647	118,241	29,135	6,752	6,325	84,364	56,177	12,800
77	728,359	266,677	162,699	132,182	32,692	7,572	7,096	94,596	62,748	14,202
78	831,705	301,745	183,789	147,912	36,603	8,494	7,954	105,997	70,034	15,771
79	944,290	341,147	207,140	165,786	40,874	9,527	8,905	118,666	78,167	17,529
80	1066,113	385,231	233,398	186,160	45,539	10,685	9,958	132,701	87,278	19,493
81	1197,174	434,531	263,316	209,365	50,725	11,987	11,134	148,202	97,500	21,683
82	1337,474	489,627	297,645	235,645	56,582	13,453	12,456	165,267	108,965	24,119
83	1487,011	551,100	337,138	265,217	63,262	15,105	13,946	183,995	121,804	26,821
84	1645,787	619,530	382,547	298,302	70,915	16,963	15,628	204,486	136,151	29,807
85	1813,801	695,497	434,624	335,118	79,692	19,048	17,524	226,837	152,136	33,098
86	1991,053	779,580	494,120	375,885	89,744	21,382	19,658	251,149	169,892	36,713
87		872,362	561,788	420,821	101,222	23,984	22,053	277,519	189,551	40,671
88		974,420	638,380	470,146	114,278	26,876	24,730	306,047	211,245	44,993
89		1086,337	724,648	524,079	129,061	30,079	27,714	336,832	235,105	49,697
90			821,343	582,840	145,722	33,624	31,036	369,972	261,265	54,802
91			929,219		164,414	37,583	34,763		289,856	
92			1049,027		185,285	42,040	38,968			
93			1181,519		208,489	47,078	43,727			
94					234,174	52,780	49,115			
95					262,492	59,228	55,206			
96					293,595	66,506	62,075			
97					327,633	74,696	69,797			
98					364,756	83,883	78,447			
99					405,116	94,149	88,100			
100						105,583	98,840			
101						118,303	110,790			
102						132,433	124,084			
103						148,096	138,854			
104						165,416	155,234			
105						184,516	173,356			
106						205,521	193,354			
107						228,554	215,360			
108						253,740	239,508			
109						281,200	265,930			

List of Figures

2.1.	Schematic drawing of the proton spin	4
2.2.	Magnetic field induced by the proton spin	4
2.3.	Alignment with an external magnetic field	4
2.4.	Precession of a proton around the axis of the main magnetic field	6
2.5.	Coordinate System representation	6
2.6.	Rotating Reference Frame	6
2.7.	RF pulse	7
2.8.	T_1 relaxation	8
2.9.	Relation between RF pulse bandwidth and slice thickness	9
2.10.	Gradient echo generation	11
2.11.	k-space image	12
2.12.	k-space coordinate system	12
2.13.	Effect of gradients in k-space	13
3.1.	FLASH sequence time course and k-space trajectory	16
3.2.	EPI sequence echo train	18
3.3.	EPI trajectory represented in k-space	18
3.4.	Time Course of a standard EPI sequence.	19
3.5.	Peano's Space Filling Curve (Iteration 3)	21
3.6.	Hilbert's Space Filling Curve (Iteration 5)	21
3.7.	Matrix indices with row major and Hilbert-Curve sorting	21
3.8.	Hilbert Grammar	23
3.9.	Hilbert's space filling curve iteration 1-3	23
3.10.	Hilbert's space filling curve iteration 5	24
3.11.	Hilbert-Moore space filling curve iteration 5	24
3.12.	TRIADS Scheme	25
3.13.	Cardiac and respiratory gating proposed by Sigfridsson	25

List of Figures

3.14. Selection order for Sigfridsson imaging scheme 26
3.15. 64 × 64 matrix sampling 32
3.16. Preface VD sampling 33
3.17. Inplace VD sampling 33
3.18. Trajectory measurement scheme 35
3.19. Gradient Amplitudes 38
3.20. Variable density time course for the Hilbert-Moore sequence 39
3.21. Phase Errors in the Hilbert-Moore sequence 40
3.22. Hilbert-Moore sequence measured trajectory 41

4.1. SMASH vs PARS reconstruction 47
4.2. Variable density autocalibrating acquisition scheme 48
4.3. GRAPPA weight calculation 49
4.4. GRAPPA reconstruction 49
4.5. MCNMLI weight calculation 50
4.6. Direct Neighborhood 52
4.7. Source and Reference selection 52
4.8. Hanning-Window 52
4.9. Simulation phantoms 53
4.10. Simulation coil set 54
4.11. Ringing-Artefacts 55
4.12. Simulation phantom with FFT Reco 55
4.13. Simulation phantom with reconstruction 55
4.14. Reconstructed and sampled k-space center 56
4.15. VD Center Sampling 56
4.16. Image quality of different start points 57
4.17. Images for best and worst start points 58
4.18. Mean absolute difference for different window sizes 60
4.19. Best window size reconstruction 61
4.20. Shepp Window Sizes 62
4.21. Sphere Phantom Field of View and Risetime 63
4.22. Sphere Phantom start point influence 65
4.23. SNR Regions 65
4.24. SNR evaluation 67

List of Figures

4.25.	Comparison between HM and EPI	68
4.26.	Volunteer brain structures overview	69
5.1.	Schematic drawing of a conventional speaker	74
5.2.	log(Amplitude) vs. Sound Pressure Level (SPL)	81
5.3.	Frequency plot comparison EPI and HM	83
5.4.	HM sequence frequencies for different TR	85
5.5.	HM sequence frequency plots for different rise times	87

List of Tables

3.1.	Amplitude and blip risetime calculation	37
4.1.	Scanner data phantom acquisition parameters	64
5.1.	Mechanisms of acoustic noise interference during fMRI	73
5.2.	Microphone calibration Sound Pressure Levels	79
5.3.	Measured SPL for main imaging sequence parameters	82
5.4.	Hilbert-Moore SPL for different FOV	83
5.5.	Hilbert-Moore SPL for different TR	84
5.6.	HM sequence SPL for different start points	86
5.7.	HM sequence SPL for different rise times	86
5.8.	SPL for single gradient axes	88
5.9.	Damped SPL for main imaging sequence parameters	89
B.1.	Calibration Tunes Lookup Table	103

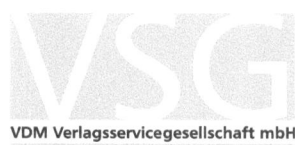

Die VDM Verlagsservicegesellschaft sucht für wissenschaftliche Verlage abgeschlossene und herausragende

Dissertationen, Habilitationen, Diplomarbeiten, Master Theses, Magisterarbeiten usw.

für die kostenlose Publikation als Fachbuch.

Sie verfügen über eine Arbeit, die hohen inhaltlichen und formalen Ansprüchen genügt, und haben Interesse an einer honorarvergüteten Publikation?

Dann senden Sie bitte erste Informationen über sich und Ihre Arbeit per Email an *info@vdm-vsg.de*.

Sie erhalten kurzfristig unser Feedback!

VDM Verlagsservicegesellschaft mbH
Dudweiler Landstr. 99
D - 66123 Saarbrücken

Telefon +49 681 3720 174
Fax +49 681 3720 1749

www.vdm-vsg.de

Die VDM Verlagsservicegesellschaft mbH vertritt

 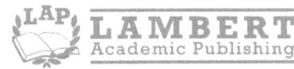 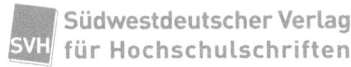

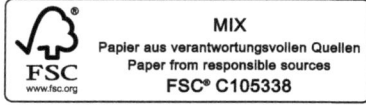

Printed by Books on Demand GmbH, Norderstedt / Germany